NEUROANATOMY RESEARCH AT THE LEADING EDGE

TYPICAL IMAGING IN ATYPICAL PARKINSON'S, SCHIZOPHRENIA, EPILEPSY AND ASYMPTOMATIC ALZHEIMER'S DISEASE

NEUROANATOMY RESEARCH AT THE LEADING EDGE

Additional books and e-books in this series can be found on Nova's website under the Series tab.

NEUROSCIENCE RESEARCH PROGRESS

Additional books and e-books in this series can be found on Nova's website under the Series tab.

NEUROANATOMY RESEARCH AT THE LEADING EDGE

TYPICAL IMAGING IN ATYPICAL PARKINSON'S, SCHIZOPHRENIA, EPILEPSY AND ASYMPTOMATIC ALZHEIMER'S DISEASE

YONGXIA ZHOU, PHD

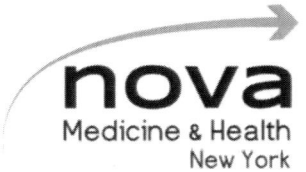

Copyright © 2021 by Nova Science Publishers, Inc.

All rights reserved. No part of this book may be reproduced, stored in a retrieval system or transmitted in any form or by any means: electronic, electrostatic, magnetic, tape, mechanical photocopying, recording or otherwise without the written permission of the Publisher.

We have partnered with Copyright Clearance Center to make it easy for you to obtain permissions to reuse content from this publication. Simply navigate to this publication's page on Nova's website and locate the "Get Permission" button below the title description. This button is linked directly to the title's permission page on copyright.com. Alternatively, you can visit copyright.com and search by title, ISBN, or ISSN.

For further questions about using the service on copyright.com, please contact:
Copyright Clearance Center
Phone: +1-(978) 750-8400   Fax: +1-(978) 750-4470   E-mail: info@copyright.com

NOTICE TO THE READER

The Publisher has taken reasonable care in the preparation of this book, but makes no expressed or implied warranty of any kind and assumes no responsibility for any errors or omissions. No liability is assumed for incidental or consequential damages in connection with or arising out of information contained in this book. The Publisher shall not be liable for any special, consequential, or exemplary damages resulting, in whole or in part, from the readers' use of, or reliance upon, this material. Any parts of this book based on government reports are so indicated and copyright is claimed for those parts to the extent applicable to compilations of such works.

Independent verification should be sought for any data, advice or recommendations contained in this book. In addition, no responsibility is assumed by the publisher for any injury and/or damage to persons or property arising from any methods, products, instructions, ideas or otherwise contained in this publication.

This publication is designed to provide accurate and authoritative information with regard to the subject matter covered herein. It is sold with the clear understanding that the Publisher is not engaged in rendering legal or any other professional services. If legal or any other expert assistance is required, the services of a competent person should be sought. FROM A DECLARATION OF PARTICIPANTS JOINTLY ADOPTED BY A COMMITTEE OF THE AMERICAN BAR ASSOCIATION AND A COMMITTEE OF PUBLISHERS.

Color graphics are available in the e-book version of this book.
All color captions are referring to e-book only.

Library of Congress Cataloging-in-Publication Data

ISBN: 978-1-53619-939-0

Published by Nova Science Publishers, Inc. † New York

Contents

Preface		**vii**
Chapter 1	Imaging Differences of Parkinson's Disease with and without Mild Cognitive Impairment	**1**
Chapter 2	Conventional Imaging Biomarkers of Atypical Parkinson's - CBS and PSP	**31**
Chapter 3	Novel Imaging Biomarkers in CBS/PSP and Asymptomatic/Symptomatic Alzheimer's	**63**
Chapter 4	Typical Imaging Biomarkers in Schizophrenia and Epilepsy	**99**
About the Author		**137**
Index		**139**

PREFACE

We had recently reported multiparametric and multi-point imaging abnormalities in mild cognitive impairment (MCI) and Parkinson's disease (PD). The prevalence rate of MCI in PD (PD-MCI) was about 20-30% and could reach 80% for long-term PD with dementia (PDD). The progression from PD-MCI to PDD incidence rate was about 11% annually, and over 90% outcome for PDD conversion after a long time (>15 years). Different from typical MCI in general Alzheimer's disease (AD-MCI), nonamnestic deficits in several cognitive domains such as executive function, attention, visual spatial and language/praxis in PD-MCI were exhibited and had been confirmed with several studies. The cognitive profile in PD-MCI could be heterogeneous including not only the typical motor disorder but also multi-domain neuropsychological problems, and might be different and more complicate than general AD-MCI. In this book, we had further demonstrated hippocampal atrophy and disrupted brain networks including default mode network (DMN) and frontoparietal network (FPN) in MCI compared to normal controls (NC) and early AD population with advanced imaging quantifications. MCI in PD, as a special case, also exhibited brain atrophy and interhemispheric dis-coordination in signature region of substantia nigra, hippocampus, anterior temporal and superior frontal cortices compared to PD without MCI. Furthermore, decreased inter-network connectivity of DMN/FPN but increased dorso-attentional network (DAN)/cerebellum/visual cortex as compensation was identified in PD-MCI using independent component analysis (ICA)-based dual regression (ICA-DR) method. Additionally, decreased global efficiency together with increased local efficiency and low-frequency synchrony of neural activity were present in PD-MCI compared to no MCI participants. As a continuing project from our previous work, these forefront results presented multi-level brain abnormalities including functional, morphological, micro-structural and molecular perspectives in MCI at early stage as well as MCI in PD, and could provide solid imaging evidence for comorbid disease diagnosis, differentiation and efficient treatment.

Corticobasal syndrome (CBS) is a rare Parkinson's symptom with abnormalities in both cortical region and basal ganglia. The neuropathology of corticobasal degeneration (CBD) includes neuronal loss, gliosis and tau deposition in the neocortex, basal ganglia and brain stem, with typical symptoms of limb apraxia, myoclonus, dystonia and alien limb. Progressive supranuclear palsy (PSP) is another atypical Parkinsonism, with supranuclear referring to the damage localized above the eye-moving centers (nuclei) in brain and palsy indicating disorder impairing eye movements. Typical brain atrophy, lower interhemispheric correlation, functional intra- and inter- network dysconnectivity patterns and structural integrity deterioration were reported in CBS and PSP patients. Specifically, cerebellum, basal ganglia, most of subcortical regions as well as cortical motor/premotor and supplementary motor areas, insula, superior frontal cortex and parietal lobe demonstrated gray matter atrophy in CBS patients compared to controls. PSP patients presented similar atrophy patterns as to CBS under resting state eyes closing (RS EC) condition, as well as during physiologically unconscious (RS PH) situation. Voxel mirrored homotopic correlation (VMHC) patterns were almost the same in CBS patients under two conditions; including lower interhemispheric correlations found in regions of motor, posterior parietal and insula, orbitofrontal, temporal lobe and visual cortex but higher VMHC in the basal ganglia such as red nucleus, hippocampus, superior frontal and cerebellum compared to controls. However, in PSP patients, predominantly higher VMHC values were present in most brain regions including frontal, occipital and parietal lobes under RS EC situation. In contrast, under the RS PH condition, similar VMHC pattern as of CBS comparing to controls was found in PSP, with a less degree of spatial spreading. Moreover, lower functional network connectivity in the superior frontal cortex, anterior cingulate cortex and anterior temporal lobe together with lower inter-network connectivity of visual-motor and frontal-cerebellum pathways were also identified in CBS patients compared to NC. And lower FPN connectivity but higher visual-motor and orbitofrontal inter-network connectivity were observed comparing PSP to CBS patients under both RS EC and RS PH conditions. Also lower mean fractional anisotropy (FA) but higher axial/radial diffusivity values were found in PSP compared to CBS in several white matter tracts including the anterior thalamic radiation, uncinate fasciculus and cingulum connecting the hippocampus based on diffusion tensor imaging (DTI), with almost identical small-worldness characteristics between two patients population. Our quantitative and multiparametric results also confirmed largely common imaging features of CBS and PSP; however, altered MRI patterns under different situations and between two patients population indicated distinct neuropathological disease mechanism.

In addition to the conventional statistical correlation map computed between time series of seed and targeted voxel/regions (static pattern), dynamic functional network connectivity (dFNC) had recently been proposed to cluster brain networks based on segmented characteristic time courses. Temporal variation and associated spatial map of all dFNC matrices could be derived using the multivariate decomposition method such as ICA and Markov modeling to obtain the most essential and informative source. State is defined as a temporal variation pattern extracted from sampled dynamic windows (segmented correlation matrices) that all participants most likely return or stay during the time course of the experiment. With advanced modeling and clustering methods, dFNC had been applied to study the functional coordination and flexibility among different networks (inter-network connectivities) for better understanding of behavior-related shifts such as vigilance/arousal and brain cognitive adaption processes. Similar to the ICA-DR modeling of multiple networks, dFNC could simplify and reveal the intrinsic and dynamic states among large-scale networks in comparison to the conventional static network analysis. The applications of these relatively new techniques in neuroscience and various diseases could help interpret brain organization and optimal integration at normal states (similar to conventional methods), as well as provide further objective and complementary information-based evidence for neuropathological confirmation. The dFNC differences were illustrated for both CBS and PSP patients under RS EC and RS PH conditions, and revealed lower temporal dynamics in PSP compared to CBS patients with shorter dwell time and less occurrence for most representative states in PSP. The results of different dynamic connectivity patterns under two RS conditions were in agreement with conventional findings of VMHC and ICA-DR as well as DTI microstructural methods reported in Chapter 2. For instance, under RS EC condition, slow dynamic transitions of salience network (SN) and central executive network (CEN) with dFNC method were consistent with the hypo-network modulation with ICA-DR algorithm in PSP compared to CBS participants. And under RS PH condition, lower SN dFNC in PSP compared to CBS were similar to the ICA-DR inter-network modulation result as well as RS EC dFNC finding. Observations of lower interhemispheric conductivity, white matter micro-structural connectivity deterioration, inter-network dis-coordination and less temporal dynamics were consistent, and indicated possible spatiotemporal dynamic communication and pathway distortion at different degrees in two patient cohorts at representative situations.

Schizophrenia is a neuropsychiatric disorder with relapsed psychosis and primary symptoms of hallucination and delusion. Gray matter atrophy in several grouped networks including thalamus, insula/anterior cingulate and postcentral gyrus had also been reported in schizophrenia. Epilepsy is a neurological disease with spontaneous and recurrent seizures caused by abnormally hyper-synchrony of neuronal activity. Precise localization of epileptic focus is important for surgical intervention, and MRI/fMRI play important role in anatomical and functional mapping of normal tissue around the lesions. Common structural brain abnormalities in both epilepsy and psychosis including diffuse brain lesions (dysgenesis) interacted with the presentation of each other, and led to the association between epilepsy and schizophrenia-like psychosis. Brain network dysfunction in the DMN, SN, visual network (VN), and CEN were identified in both patient groups. Conventional imaging results demonstrated significant gray matter atrophy, VMHC deficits, lower regional homogeneity pattern, static intra- and inter- network dysconnectivity as well as lower fractional amplitude of low frequency fluctuation (fALFF) activities with different regional weighting and significance in two patient cohorts. Based on the results of dFNC, reversal patterns in each state of both patient cohorts with less overall dynamics such as shorter dwell time and lower occurrence frequency compared to controls were demonstrated. The general inter-network hypo-connectivity pattern with reduced numbers of transitions, less dwell time in majorities of states with a dip plateau form were present in epilepsy compared to schizophrenia. These anti-phase synchronization and dis-coordination between neuronal networks in both patients were likely due to injured thalamus and dorsolateral prefrontal regions (executive control dysfunction) in schizophrenia, and thalamic-related hippocampal sclerosis or brain lesions in critical temporal lobe hubs that were in charge of brain wave generation and persistence in epilepsy. Our results were consistent with previous dFNC findings that epilepsy patients tend to stay in more negative and static brain states, while schizophrenia group tend to switch between positive and negative states and both groups showing different paces or asynchronous brain waves than controls.

Taken together, we had analyzed imaging abnormalities of a special case of PD with MCI (comorbid motor and dementia disorder), two rare cases of PD-CBS and PSP, as well as two neuropsychiatric/neurological diseases including schizophrenia and epilepsy in this new book. Relatively novel dFNC and regional homogeneity methods together with the conventional imaging metrics such as ICA-DR, VMHC, fALFF, voxel-based morphometry (VBM) and graph-theory based small-worldness were implemented to investigate the full-spectrum quantitative features of these disorders. Conductivity and neuronal circuit alterations under different situations such as resting state with eyes closing or physiologically unconsciousness in CBS and PSP, as well as dynamic state-based parametric commons/differences between two disease models such as schizophrenia and epilepsy provided complementary and confirmative imaging evidence for more accurate disease diagnosis. Our comprehensive results were in agreement with previous work, revealing reliable and systematic, voxel-wise and network-based, static and transit, unique and integrative quantifications for better interpretation of the underlying disease mechanism and early prevention. The aim of this book is thus intended to provide readers some new insights of applying various imaging techniques to more accurately diagnose and distinguish each subtype and rare/comorbid cases of several brain disorders. The specific and combined imaging features utilized that could pinpoint the exact abnormalities of these atypical and/or rare diseases are the highlights of this new book. This book would hope to convey the technical development and application of cutting-edge and advanced imaging methods in special and challenging brain diseases. The author would like to acknowledge the Alzheimer's disease neuroimaging initiative (ADNI) center and NeuroImaging Tools & Resources Collaboratory (NITRC) database for providing valuable original imaging data.

Specifically, Chapter 1 covered the topics of multiparametric imaging differences for PD with MCI compared to PD without MCI utilizing typical imaging methods including VBM, VMHC, fALFF, DTI and ICA-DR. Neuroimaging results of general MCI such as hippocampal subfields shrinkage in MCI and AD as well as DMN sub-network risk factor increments together with ICA-DR algorithm were illustrated additionally. Differentiation of two subtypes of atypical Parkinson's disease- CBS and PSP with conventional and advanced imaging comparisons under two resting state conditions (RS EC and RS PH) were demonstrated in Chapter 2. Further exploration of relatively new methods such as dFNC and regional homogeneity were investigated in Chapter 3 for the same CBS and PSP groups. Correlations between PET amyloid accumulation and MRI regional volumetry in asymptomatic AD were investigated, in addition to the cerebral blood flow alterations and association with the clinical composite scores in AD. As another example of dFNC application, Chapter 4 elucidated the dynamic network changes as well as the underlying mechanism in schizophrenia and epilepsy patients together with the conventional imaging results. Commons and differences of imaging results in two patient cohorts were then discussed and summarized.

Chapter 1 – We had reported multiple imaging abnormalities in different subtypes of mild cognitive impairment (MCI) such as early MCI (EMCI), late MCI and early probable Alzheimer's disease (pAD) using unique multiomic features together with the distinct disease profile of each neurodegenerative disease in our previous work. The purposes of this study are to: 1. investigate further the functional and structural differences in MCI data cohort in addition to the summaries of previous related neuroimaging findings; and 2. illustrate the subtle differences in MCI compared to no MCI subtypes in Parkinson's disease (PD) with advanced imaging metrics such as intra-/inter- network connectivities and sub-band functional activity as well as systematic small-worldness analysis.

Our imaging results had demonstrated hippocampal atrophy and disrupted brain networks including default mode network (DMN) and frontoparietal network (FPN) in MCI compared to normal controls (NC) and early AD population with advanced imaging quantifications. MCI in PD (PD-MCI), as a special case, also exhibited brain atrophy and interhemispheric dis-coordination in typical regions of substantia nigra, hippocampus, anterior temporal and superior frontal cortices compared to PD without MCI. Furthermore, decreased inter-network connectivity of DMN/FPN but increased dorsal attentional network/cerebellum as compensation was identified in PD-MCI with decreased global efficiency together with increased local efficiency and low-frequency synchrony. These consistent results presented multi-level brain abnormalities including functional, morphological, micro-structural and molecular perspectives in MCI at early stage as well as MCI in PD, and could provide solid imaging evidence for comorbid disease prevention and efficient treatment.

Chapter 2 – We had applied advanced MRI and PET neuroimaging techniques in various neurodegenerative diseases such as functional coordination and inter-network connectivity in typical PD and comorbid PD with MCI patients previously. The purposes of this study are to: 1. reveal the imaging differences in corticobasal degeneration (CBD) and progressive supranuclear palsy (PSP) compared to controls as well as the differences between these two sub-types; 2. investigate brain alterations with imaging data acquired under different conditions in two patient cohorts; and 3. perform comprehensive analysis such as tract-based structural connectivity and graph-theory based small-worldness as well as correlations among different neuroimaging metrics.

Typical brain atrophy, lower interhemispheric correlation, functional intra- and inter- dysconnectivity patterns and structural integrity deterioration were reported in CBS and PSP patients. Specifically, cerebellum, basal ganglia, most of subcortical regions and cortical motor/premotor and supplementary motor areas, insula, superior frontal cortex and parietal lobe demonstrated gray matter atrophy in CBS/CBD patients compared to normal controls (NC). PSP patients presented similar atrophy patterns as to CBS under resting state eyes closing (RS EC) condition, as well as during resting state physiologically unconscious (RS PH) situation. Comparing PSP to CBS under two conditions, gray matter atrophy in the cerebellum, visual cortex and striatum, but more gray matter density in the cortical parietal, scattered temporal, thalamus and superior frontal regions were present. VMHC patterns were similar in CBS patients compared to controls under resting state eyes closing and physiologically unconscious conditions, including lower interhemispheric correlations found in regions of motor, posterior parietal and insula, orbitofrontal, temporal lobe and visual cortices but higher VMHC in the basal ganglia such as red nucleus, hippocampus, superior frontal and cerebellum. However in PSP patients, predominantly higher VMHC were present in most brain regions including frontal, occipital and parietal lobes under RS EC situation. In contrast, under the RS PH condition, similar VMHC pattern as of CBS comparing to controls was found in PSP, with a less degree of spatial spreading. Lower functional network connectivity in the superior frontal cortex, anterior cingulate cortex and anterior temporal lobe together with lower inter-network connectivity of visual-motor and frontal-cerebellum pathways were identified in CBS patients compared to NC. Lower frontoparietal network connectivity but higher visual-motor and orbitofrontal inter-network connectivity were observed comparing PSP to CBS patients under two resting state conditions. Also lower mean FA but higher axial/radial diffusivity values were found in PSP compared to CBS groups in several white matter tracts such as anterior thalamic radiation, uncinate fasciculus and cingulum connecting the hippocampus, with similar small-worldness characteristics between two patients population. Our comprehensive results also confirmed largely common imaging features of CBS and PSP; however, altered MRI patterns under different situations and between two patients population indicated distinct neuropathological disease mechanism.

Chapter 3 – There have been numerous studies investigating improvement of pattern recognition and revealing the underlying temporal dynamics in large-scale networks with more adaptive and better-characterized methods such as dynamic functional network connectivity (dFNC) algorithm. The specific objectives of this chapter are to: 1. explore further dFNC differences between two atypical PD groups -CBS and PSP under two resting state (RS) conditions, in addition to conventional imaging findings in Chapter 2; and 2. introduce as well as analyze some other novel imaging data such as cerebral blood flow with arterial spin labeling technique and PET/MRI correlation in early and asymptomatic Alzheimer's disease (AD).

Our results demonstrated dFNC differences between CBS and PSP under both resting state eyes closing (RS EC) and physiological unconsciousness (RS PH) conditions and confirmed the lower temporal dynamics in PSP compared to CBS patients. For instance, under RS EC condition, both lower salience network (SN) and central executive network (CEN) dynamic transition with dFNC method and hypo-network modulation with ICA-DR algorithm were in agreement in PSP compared to CBS participants. Also under RS PH condition, lower SN dFNC in PSP compared to CBS were similar to the ICA-DR inter-network modulation result as well as RS EC dFNC finding. Disruption of SN dynamics under both RS conditions was probably related to the disinhibition function that was common to both PD subtypes and state-shifting role of SN. Observations of lower interhemispheric conductivity, white matter microstructural connectivity deterioration, inter-network dis-coordination and less temporal dynamics were consistent, indicating possible spatiotemporal communication and pathway distortion at different degrees in two patient cohorts. Moreover, we found significantly lower cerebral blood flow (CBF) values measured with MRI arterial spin labeling (ASL) technique in MCI/AD patients compared to controls ($P < 0.05$) for most regions, with a lower trend in AD compared to MCI. Strong correlations between CBF and memory composite score were present more in controls, less in MCI and AD patients; and CBF in a few regions correlated with language composite score only in AD. Also significant associations between amyloid deposition in the anterior cingulate/orbito-medial prefrontal regions and MRI temporoparietal volume were identified in asymptomatic Aβ+ carriers. The combination of these novel imaging metrics such as dFNC and ASL-CBF together with conventional imaging quantifications could improve disease detection accuracy and validate multiparametric metrics with better interpretation.

Chapter 4 – Imaging abnormalities in schizophrenia and epilepsy had been reported with several metrics previously, systematic and integrative analyses are needed for better diseases diagnosis and treatment. The purposes of this chapter are to: 1. apply the relatively new dynamic functional network connectivity (dFNC) and regional homogeneity (ReHo) analyses to both schizophrenia and epilepsy patients; 2. reveal the conventional imaging differences in these two patient cohorts compared to controls with VBM, VMHC, fALFF, ReHo, ICA-DR and small-worldness methods; and 3. Investigate further the commons and differences of two diseases based on comprehensive imaging findings.

Regarding the results of dFNC, reversal patterns in each state of both patient cohorts with less overall dynamics compared to controls were demonstrated. The general inter-network hypo-connectivity pattern with reduced numbers of transitions, less dwell time in majorities of states with a dip plateau form were present in epilepsy compared to schizophrenia. Conventional imaging results demonstrated significant gray matter atrophy, VMHC deficits, lower regional homogeneity pattern, static intra- and inter- network dysconnectivities as well as lower fALFF activities with different regional weighting and significance levels in two patient cohorts. Our results utilizing both conventional and relatively novel methods were in agreement with previous work, providing reliable and systematic, voxel-wise and network-based, static and dynamic, unique and multiparametric perspectives for revealing the underlying disease mechanism with accurate specifications.

Chapter 1

IMAGING DIFFERENCES OF PARKINSON'S DISEASE WITH AND WITHOUT MILD COGNITIVE IMPAIRMENT

ABSTRACT

We had reported multiple imaging abnormalities in different subtypes of mild cognitive impairment (MCI) such as early MCI (EMCI), late MCI and early probable Alzheimer's disease (pAD) using unique multiomic features together with the distinct disease profile of each subtype in our previous work. The purposes of this study are to: 1. investigate further the functional and structural differences in MCI data cohort in addition to the summaries of previous related neuroimaging findings; and 2. illustrate the subtle differences in MCI compared to no MCI subtypes in Parkinson's disease (PD) with advanced imaging metrics such as intra-/inter- network connectivities and sub-band functional activity as well as systematic small-worldness analysis.

Our imaging results had demonstrated hippocampal atrophy and disrupted brain networks including default mode network (DMN) and frontoparietal network (FPN) in MCI compared to normal controls (NC) and early AD population with advanced imaging quantifications. MCI in PD (PD-MCI), as a special case, also exhibited brain atrophy and interhemispheric dis-coordination in typical regions of substantia nigra, hippocampus, anterior temporal and superior frontal cortices compared to PD without MCI. Furthermore, decreased inter-network connectivity of DMN/FPN but increased dorsal attentional network/cerebellum as compensation was identified in PD-MCI with decreased global efficiency together with increased local efficiency and low-frequency synchrony. These consistent results presented multi-level brain abnormalities including functional, morphological, micro-structural and molecular perspectives in MCI at early stage as well as MCI in PD, and could provide solid imaging evidence for comorbid disease prevention and efficient treatment.

Keywords: dual regression, independent component analysis, voxel-mirrored homotopic correlation, interhemispheric conductivity, mild cognitive impairment, Parkinson's disease, efficiency, functional connectivity, brain atrophy, voxel-based morphometry, functional activity, resting-state functional connectivity, fractional amplitude of low frequency fluctuation, early MCI, probable AD, hippocampus, subfield segmentation, default mode network, frontoparietal network, functional compensation

1. INTRODUCTION

In multi-domain (MD)-mild cognitive impairment (MCI) including MCI in Parkinson's disease (PD-MCI), the cut-off Montreal cognitive assessment (MoCA) score with range ≥19/20 and ≤26/27 was well-documented [1, 2]. Acceptable accuracy for MoCA and even superior to the Mini-mental state examination (MMSE) for MD-MCI and PD-MCI detection had been reported. These cut-off points for MD-MCI were slightly higher than the simple MCI assessment (24/25 for age 60-79 group) and comparable to standard MMSE score [3, 4]. The prevalence rate of MCI in PD was about 20-30% and long-term PD with dementia (PDD) could reach 80% [2]. In addition, another study also reported an overall of 25% conversion to PD-MCI from normal cognition in PD (PD-NC or PD-noMCI) [5]. The progression from PD-MCI to PDD incidence rate was about 11% annually, and over 90% outcome for PDD conversion after a long time (>15 years) [6]. Different from typical MCI in general Alzheimer's disease (AD-MCI), nonamnestic deficits in several cognitive domains such as executive function, attention, visual spatial and language/praxis in PD-MCI were exhibited and had been confirmed with many studies [7-9]. The cognitive profile in PD-MCI could be heterogeneous including not only the typical motor disorder but also multi-domain neuropsychological problems, and might be different and more complicate than typical AD-MCI [10-11].

For neuroimaging findings using functional connectivity with MRI (fcMRI), decreased default mode network (DMN), especially within the medial prefrontal cortex (MPFC) as well as between MPFC and posterior cingulate cortex (PCC) were identified in PD-MCI compared to PD-noMCI [12-14]. Furthermore, lower fcMRI values between hippocampus and inferior frontal gyrus (IFG), between PCC and inferior parietal lobe (IPL), as well as between anterior temporal lobe and IFG comparing PD-MCI to PD-noMCI were demonstrated [15]. On a microstructural level with diffusion tensor imaging (DTI), PD patients demonstrated lower fractional anisotropy (FA) in the substantia nigra middle portion compared to normal controls [16]. And higher radial diffusivity was observed in frontal areas in PD before MCI with earlier onset compared to PD-no MCI; both having white matter integrity change such as demyelination in the critical areas in general PD population [14]. The PDD participants had decreased volume in the corpus callosum compared to PD-MCI and controls, also the callosal DTI-FA in segments connecting fronto-striatal and posterior brain regions was correlated with cognitive performance in PD patients [17, 18]. As previously reported, depleted dopamine in the striatum including caudate and putamen were related to the attention and memory deficits in PD [19]. In addition, the caudate dopamine transporter levels together with clinical scores, cerebrospinal fluid (CSF) Aβ42 concentration, depression scale and eye movement questionnaire could predict cognitive impairment in PD [20].

Based on electroencephalogram (EEG) measurements, lower EEG entropy at baseline and background rhythm frequency, higher the probability of cognitive decline and larger hazard ratio for developing dementia in PD were found [21-22]. Quantitative EEG (qEEG) analyses such as spectrum and connectivity could be used to detect subtle cognitive impairment in PD, identify risk factors and stage disease severity. These techniques had been used for longitudinal monitoring and performance prediction as well as early prevention and later-stage evaluation [23-27]. EEG had also been implemented for therapeutic assessments including donepezil treatment for PD-MCI and rehabilitation strategy for neurological diseases with tomography and multimodal neurophysiology integration [28-29].

We had previously reported multiple imaging abnormalities in different subtypes of MCI such as early MCI (EMCI), late MCI and early probable AD (pAD) using several unique imaging and multiomic features together with the distinct disease profile of each neurodegenerative disease [16, 30, 31]. The purposes of this study are to: 1. investigate further the functional and structural differences of the MCI data cohort in addition to certain summaries of previous related findings; and 2. illustrate the subtle differences in PD-MCI compared to PD-no MCI subtypes with advanced imaging metrics such as intra- and inter- network connectivities, sub-band functional activity as well as graph-theory based systematic analyses.

2. METHODS

2.1. Data Acquisitions and Processing in General MCI Data Cohort

MRI/PET Imaging data used in the preparation of this article were obtained from the ADNI database (http://ida.loni.usc.edu). The primary goal of ADNI has been to test whether serial MRI, positron emission tomography (PET), other biological markers, and clinical and neuropsychological assessment can be combined to measure the progression of mild cognitive impairment (MCI) and early Alzheimer's disease (AD). ADNI is the result of efforts of many co-investigators from a broad range of academic institutions and private corporations, and subjects have been recruited from over 50 sites across the United States and Canada. For up-to-date information, see www.adni-info.org.

For the general MCI study, the MCI and normal control (NC) images from our previous reported ADNI data cohort were further analyzed with the relatively new independent component analysis with dual regression (ICA-DR) method for intra-/inter- network connectivity and pattern remapping computation. The ICA-DR network templates included not only conventional hubs such as DMN, motor, visual and thalamocortical connectivity patterns, but also typical and relevant brain status circuits such as frontoparietal network (FPN) and dorso-attentional network (DAN) [16]. Additionally, illustrations of the hippocampal subfields volumetry, fcMRI maps and DMN sub-network weighted scaling factor for risk evaluation together with comparisons between MCI and NC/early AD groups as well as longitudinal prediction and correlation were demonstrated with the data introduced in our previous work [30, 31]. Volumetry of hippocampus including the total intracranial volume (ICV) and seven main subfields, such as cornu ammonis (CA) subfield 1 (CA1), CA2, CA3, CA4, dentate gyrus (DG) and subiculum (SUB) were compared between three groups including EMCI, pAD and NC. The multiple DMN sub-network functional connectivity regulation factors consisted of 11 metrics calculated based on the weighted inter-module normalization fractions from six sub-networks of DMN such as weighted posterior by ventral DMN (WPDMN_to_WVDMN) and weighted anterior-dorsal DMN (WADDMN) by median value (WADDMN_MEDIAN), four symmetric sub-networks and one total network failure quotient (NFQ) quantification values [31].

2.2. PD-MCI Participants, Imaging Parameters and Post-Processing

For the PD-MCI data cohort, all participants were recruited and managed in the Parkinson's Progression Markers Initiative (PPMI) program as one featured ADNI center that contains and manages the full set of imaging and clinical data. Available and most recent fMRI imaging data were downloaded and processed [16]. The unified Parkinson's disease rating scale (UPDRS) score was obtained from all participants for assessing motor and tremor related function. The MoCA score was collected, and cut-off of 21-27 points were used for PD with MCI and range of 28-30 were for PD without MCI symptom [2].

Table 1. Demographic information of subjects in two sub-groups of the PD data cohort including PD with MCI and without MCI.
The MoCA score was significantly lower in PD with MCI group than PD without MCI group (P = 0.025). The UPDRS score was slightly higher in PD with MCI group but no significant difference between two sub-groups (P = 0.368)

Group	Age (Years)	Women n/ %	Total N	UPDRS	MoCA
PD-MCI	70.8 ± 3.6	1/ 20%	5	35.6 ± 5.6	24.8 ± 1.2
PD-No MCI	64.8 ± 2.9	5/ 36%	14	29.7 ± 2.2	28.9 ± 0.2
P-value	0.218			0.368	0.025

As listed in Table 1, resting-state (RS)-fMRI data from 14 PD patients without MCI (age: 64.8 ± SD 2.9 years, UPDRS score = 29.7 ± 2.2, 5 women, MoCA score = 28.9 ± 0.2 with range of 28-30), and 5 PD with MCI patients (age: 70.8 ± 3.6 years, UPDRS score = 35.6 ± 5.6, 1 women, MoCA score = 24.8 ± 1.2 with range of 21-27) were processed further. Significantly lower MoCA score was found in PD with MCI group compared to PD without MCI group (P = 0.025), with trend of higher UPDRS score in PD-MCI group.

All MRI experiments were performed using the 3T scanner with standardized imaging protocols. For the resting-state (RS)-fMRI data, a standard gradient-echo EPI sequence (TR/TE = 2400/25 msec, flip angle = 80°, number of volumes = 210, spatial resolution = 3.3 x 3.3 x 5.0 mm^3) was performed. The 3D MPRAGE (TR/TI/TE = 2300/900/2.9 ms, flip angle = 9°, matrix size = 256 x 256 x 176, resolution = 1 x 1x 1 mm^3) was also obtained for structural and morphological analysis such as gray matter atrophy, as well as the reference image and anatomical normalization of seed-based fMRI functional connectivity and coordination data.

The MRI and fMRI images were processed with in-house developed scripts to derive the voxel-mirrored homotopic correlation (VMHC), voxel-based morphometry (VBM), ICA-DR, multiple seeds-based resting-state functional connectivity (RSFC) patterns and fractional amplitude of low frequency fluctuation (fALFF) maps, as described in details from our previous works [16, 30, 31]. Between-group comparisons of quantitative post-processed images were performed with advanced statistical tools using FMRIB Software Library (FSL, http://www.fmrib.ox.ac.uk/fsl) toolbox. Graph theory based small-worldness systematic analysis was performed to the fcMRI data with correlation matrix generated from 116 seeds-based RSFC, and statistical comparison results between PD-MCI and no MCI sub-groups for all metrics were derived finally.

3. RESULTS

3.1. Comparisons between General MCI, Early AD and NC

Except the slightly higher intracranial volume in EMCI compared to NC, the subfield volumetry in Figure 1A demonstrated significant and gradual hippocampal atrophy in early probable AD compared to EMCI and NC ($P < 0.05$) for several subfields, including bilateral CA1, DG and CA as well as left BA35 and total volume. The most significant atrophy subfields were in the CA1 and DG with $P < 10^{-7}$ comparing early probable AD to NC; and also in the DG/CA1 comparing EMCI to NC ($P < 0.002$). In addition, significantly higher DMN NFQ risk factors in pAD compared to EMCI ($P = 0.02$) and NC ($P = 0.01$) were identified in Figure 1B. Several higher sub-network connectivity risk factors including WADDMN_MEDIAN and WPDMN_to_WVDMN ratios in pAD compared to NC ($P \leq 0.02$) were present as well, together with higher WADDMN_MEDIAN factor comparing pAD to EMCI ($P = 0.007$) but lower weighted ventro WVDMN_to_WADDMN ratio ($P = 0.01$).

Based on the ICA-DR algorithm, altered temporal, FPN, DMN and sensorimotor network connectivities were observed in MCI compared to

NC groups (Figure 2, P < 0.001). Examples of three sub-network connectivity of DMN and FPN were demonstrated in Figure 3 and Figure 4 respectively. Figure 3 of ICA-DR based three DMN sub-networks showed decreased posterior intra-DMN (posterior cingulate) as well as inter-DMN-FPN and temporal connectivities, but increased frontal intra-DMN (medial prefrontal cortex) connectivities together with higher inter- DMN-basal ganglia and motor/supplementary motor/somatosensory connections in MCI compared to NC groups were observed. And Figure 4 of three FPN sub-networks exhibited decreased intra-FPN as well as inter- FPN and temporal/insular/DMN/thalamus/orbitofrontal network connectivities in MCI compared to NC. On the other hand, increased inter- FPN and motor/supplementary motor network /visual precuneus connectivities in MCI patients existed as well.

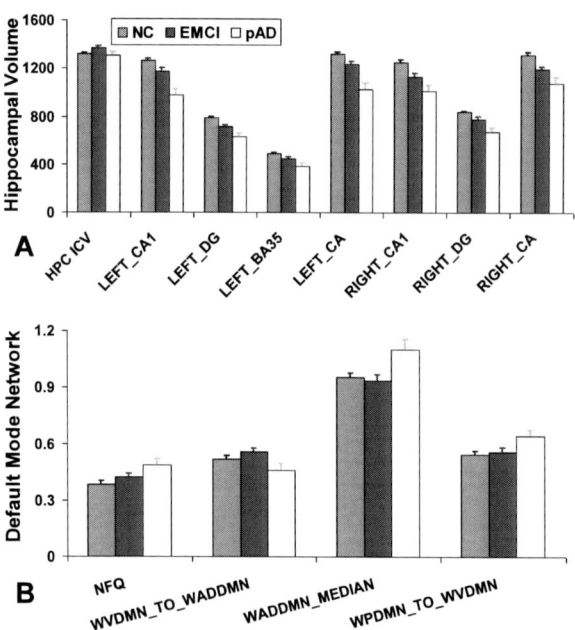

Figure 1. Significant differences of hippocampal subfield volume and DMN subnetwork metrics in three patient population (P < 0.05). A: Reduction of hippocampal subfield volume in early MCI and pAD compared to controls. B: Increased DMN sub-network connectivity risk factor (NFQ) in pAD compared to MCI and NC.

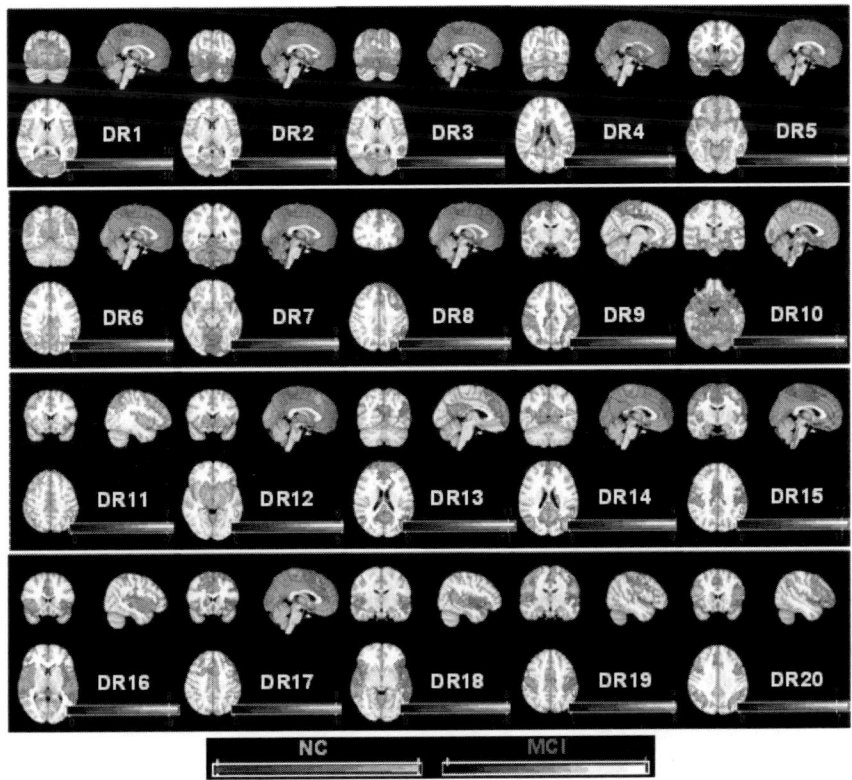

Figure 2. ICA-DR components identified in general EMCI and NC groups (P < 0.001). Blue-Green for control group (NC) and overlapped with the red-orange color for MCI group. Altered temporal, FPN, DMN and sensorimotor network connectivities could be appreciated in MCI compared to NC groups. Ten categories of representative ICA-DR components for initial template matching and 2nd-level dual regression remapping [16] were: 1) DR1, DR2, DR3: visual networks consisting of several sub-networks of different regions such as lingual, calcarine, precuneus and cuneus 2) DR4, DR10, DR12: thalamocortical networks with visual, cerebellum, temporal and frontal sub-networks 3) DR5: corticostriatal network including caudate, medial orbitofrontal and anterior temporal regions 4) DR6, DR13, DR14: posterior, anterior portions and typical whole DMN 5) DR7: cerebellum and basal ganglia 6) DR8, DR11, DR20: left, right and whole fronto-parietal networks (FPN) 7) DR9, DR15, DR19: motor, sensory and supplementary motor networks 8) DR16: auditory cortex, insula and anterior cingulate (salience network) 9) DR17: frontal network including dorsolateral prefrontal cortex (DLPFC) and DAN 10) DR18: temporal network including inferior parietal lobe.

As reported in our recent work, comparing general MCI to controls, patients had decreased hippocampal fcMRI in the temporal cortex including hippocampus, hypothalamus and medial prefrontal cortex [30].

However, increased fcMRI in the cerebellum, dorso-lateral prefrontal cortex (DLPFC), superior parietal and supplementary motor regions (Figure 5; P < 0.01) were observed as well. Another typical network-DMN fcMRI comparison identified similar pattern of lower fcMRI in the bilateral hippocampus, medial prefrontal cortex and posterior cingulate in MCI patients, but higher fcMRI in the DLPFC, orbitofrontal cortex, superior parietal and inferior temporal regions.

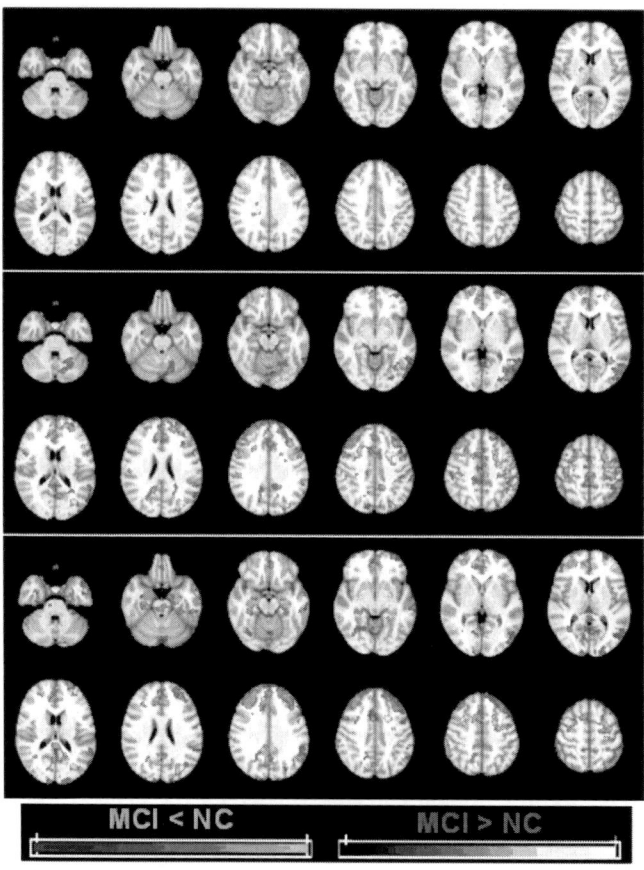

Figure 3. Decreased posterior intra-DMN (posterior cingulate), inter- DMN-FPN and temporal connectivities (blue color) was demonstrated, together with increased connections in the frontal intra-DMN (medial prefrontal cortex) as well as inter- DMN-basal ganglia and motor/supplementary motor/somatosensory areas (red color) in MCI compared to NC groups, based on three ICA-DR DMN sub-network components (P <0.001).

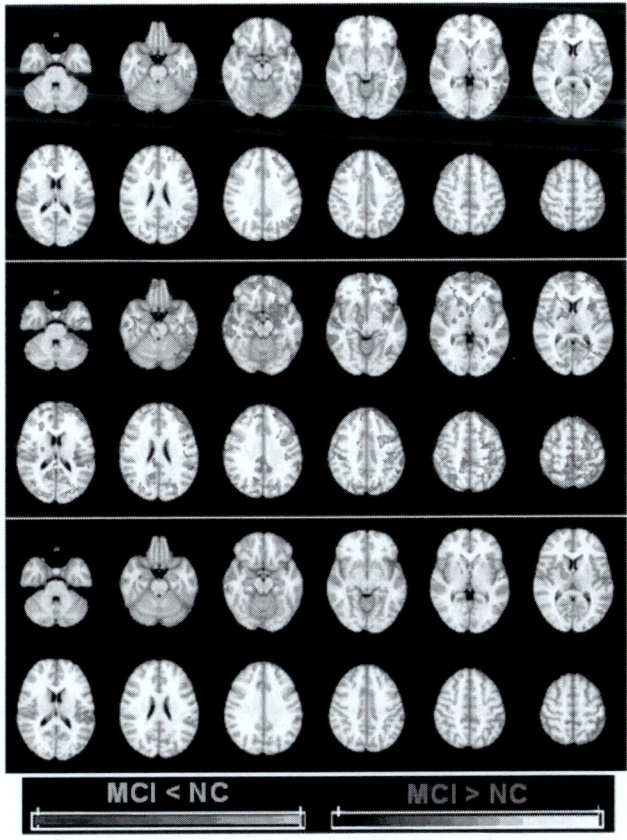

Figure 4. Decreased intra-FPN as well as inter- FPN and temporal/insular/DMN/ thalamus/orbitofrontal network connectivities (blue color) in MCI compared to NC groups with three ICA-DR FPN sub-networks. Increased inter- FPN and motor/supplementary motor network /visual precuneus connections in MCI patients (red color) existed as well ($P < 0.001$).

Furthermore, as indicated in another of our recent works [31], longitudinal change of molecular tau burden was predicted by baseline tau and amyloid level as displayed in Figure 6. For instance, significant correlations ($P < 0.01$) between longitudinal changes of tau tangle deposition and baseline tau in several brain regions such as left hippocampus, middle temporal region, superior frontal and parietal cortices, post-central area, cuneus and precuneus, parsorbitalis and rostral middle frontal area were observed in Figure 6A [31]. And baseline amyloid accumulation also predicted longitudinal tau change with significant correlations (P < 0.01) in multiple brain regions such as bilateral temporal cortices including hippocampus, fusiform, lingual, lateral occipital, postcentral, parietal, pericalcarine, paracentral, supramarginal and orbitofrontal cortices (Figure 6B).

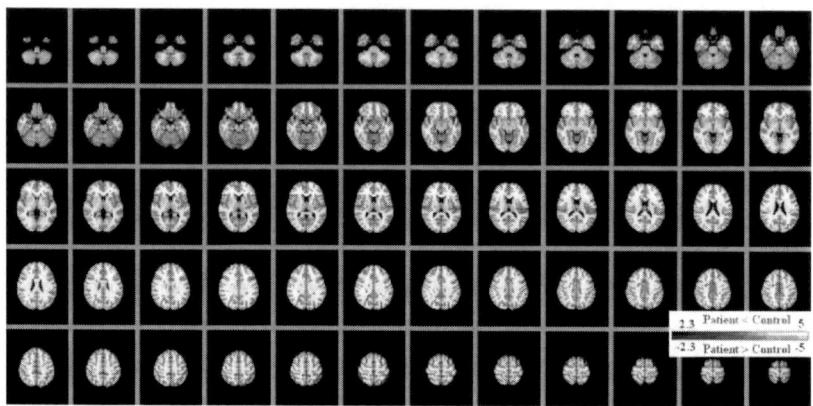

Figure 5. fcMRI from hippocampus and comparison between MCI and NC (P < 0.01) Adapted from [30], Use with Permission.

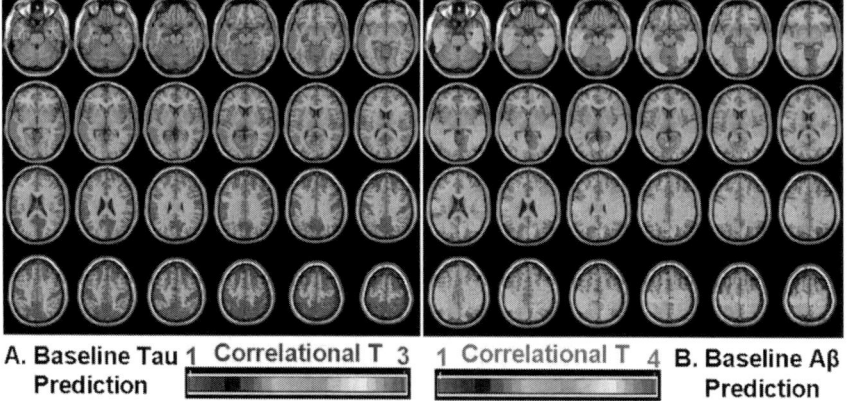

Figure 6. Longitudinal change of molecular tau burden predicted by baseline tau and amyloid level for all participants in numerous brain regions. A: Significant correlation (P < 0.01) between longitudinal tau change and baseline tau deposition in brain regions such as left hippocampus, middle and inferior temporal regions, superior frontal and parietal cortices, post-central area, cuneus and precuneus, parsorbitalis and rostral middle frontal area. B: Baseline amyloid accumulation also predicted longitudinal tau change with significant correlations (P < 0.01) in regions such as bilateral temporal cortices including hippocampus, fusiform, lingual, lateral occipital, postcentral, parietal, pericalcarine, paracentral, supramarginal and orbitofrontal cortices. Adapted from [31], use with permission.

3.2. Comparisons between PD-MCI and PD-No MCI

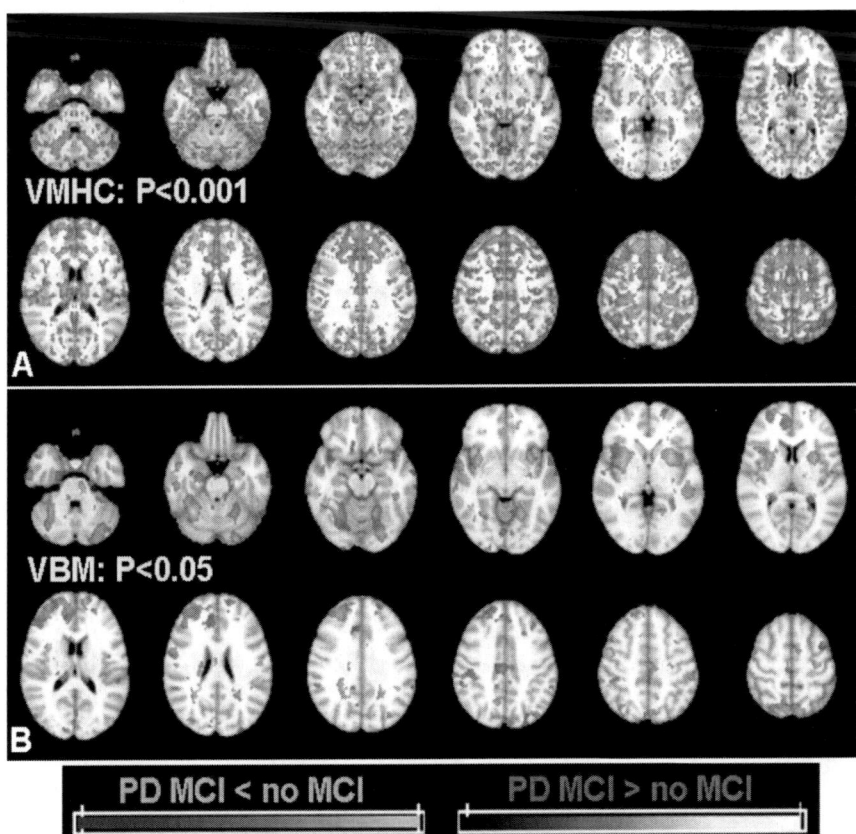

Figure 7. A: VMHC differences comparing PD with MCI to PD without MCI (P < 0.001); blue for PD-MCI < no MCI and red for PD-MCI > no MCI. Decreased VMHC in the basal ganglia including substantia nigra swallow tail signature sign of PD, hippocampus, anterior temporal and frontal regions, superior parietal, caudate and thalamus were observed in PD-MCI compared to no MCI groups (blue color). While increased VMHC in the visual cortex, orbitofrontal and inferior parietal regions were found as well (red). B: VBM results showed decreased gray matter density (atrophy) in the hippocampus, insular, anterior temporal and superior frontal cortices, superior parietal regions together with motor and supplementary motor areas in PD with MCI patients compared to no MCI group (blue). A few clusters in the cerebellum, lingual/cuneus and premotor presented higher gray matter density in PD with MCI instead (red color).

Figure 7A showed the VMHC differences comparing PD with MCI to PD without MCI groups with significant results at P < 0.001. Decreased

VMHC in the basal ganglia including the swallow tail sign of the substantia nigra, hippocampus, anterior temporal and frontal regions, superior parietal cluster, precentral, lateral occipital, central opercularis, caudate and thalamus were observed in PD-MCI. While increased VMHC values in the occipital pole, orbito- and superior- frontal and inferior parietal regions were found in PD-MCI sub-group additionally.

Table 2. Significant VMHC differences comparing PD-MCI to PD-no MCI sub-groups with P < 0.001. Brain clusters on one side are listed due to the symmetrical interhemispheric computation, with size and maximal centroid voxel (vox) information

Brain Clusters	Cluster Size	P-value	MAX Z score	MAX X(vox)	MAX Y(vox)	MAX Z(vox)
A. Regions showing decreased VMHC in PD-MCI compared to PD-no MCI (P < 0.001)						
Fusiform gyrus	4003	0	11.5	61	29	27
Cerebellum	865	1.29E-25	13.3	41	76	27
Lateral occipital cortex	315	1.45E-12	8.92	60	18	22
Superior temporal gyrus	226	7.19E-10	8.71	22	63	25
Frontal pole	189	1.20E-08	9.89	30	84	55
Precentral gyrus	187	1.41E-08	11.2	57	53	72
Caudate	148	3.58E-07	6.86	38	71	35
Supramarginal gyrus	144	4.77E-07	9.5	11	48	49
Medial frontal gyrus	140	6.56E-07	7.53	34	87	34
Temporal pole	110	1.01E-05	10.8	33	71	21
Central opercular cortex	102	2.17E-05	7.48	24	67	42
Inferior frontal gyrus	94	4.74E-05	7.92	59	80	44
Parahippocampus	76	0.00030	6.53	62	47	24
Brain stem	68	0.00071	7	48	43	11
B. Regions showing increased VMHC in PD-MCI compared to PD-no MCI (P < 0.001)						
Superior frontal gyrus	29594	0	17.4	41	70	66
Occipital pole	79	0.000219	10.9	37	11	37

Quantitative brain clusters showing significant differences of VMHC between two groups (P < 0.001) are listed in Table 2. Figure 7B identified decreased gray matter density (atrophy) in the hippocampus, anterior temporal and superior frontal cortices, insular, superior parietal cluster together with precentral motor and supplementary motor areas were found in PD with MCI patients compared to PD without MCI group (P < 0.05). On the other hand, a few clusters in the cerebellum, lingual, cuneus and premotor presented higher gray matter density in PD with MCI.

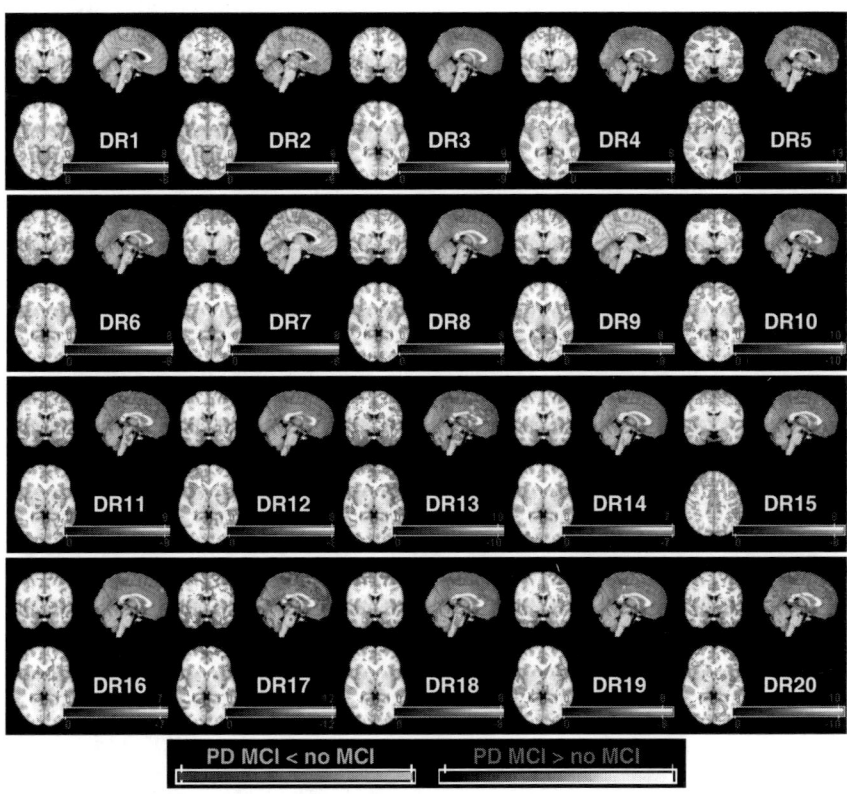

Figure 8. ICA-DR differences between PD with MCI and without MCI (P < 0.001).

The 20 ICA-DR components comparing the intra- and inter-network differences between PD with MCI and without MCI were demonstrated in Figure 8 for 3D view and Figures 9&10 for multi-slice 2D view for early 10 and later 10 components respectively (all with P < 0.001). The ICA-DR identified altered network connectivities in the temporal cortex, FPN, medial prefrontal cortex, insular, anterior cingulate cortex, motor area and basal ganglia together with DMN/DAN such as decreased medial prefrontal-temporal connectivity, with increased visual, cerebellum and

DAN connection including DLPFC in PD-MCI compared to no MCI sub-groups.

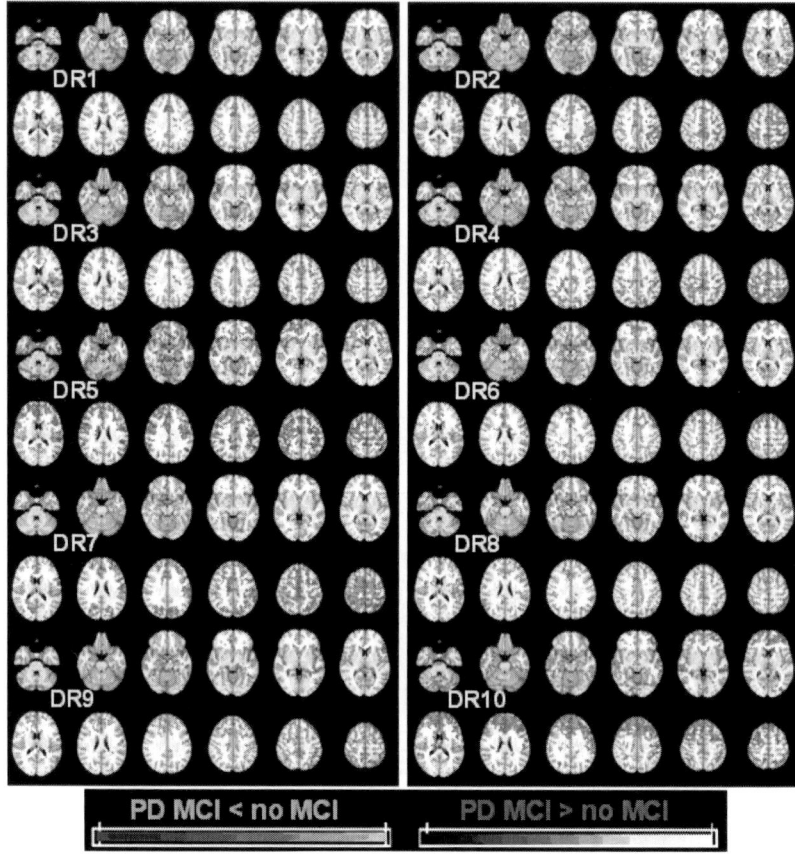

Figure 9. ICA-DR algorithm identified altered network connectivity in the temporal cortex, FPN, thalamus, medial prefrontal cortex and DMN/DAN such as decreased medial prefrontal-temporal connectivity (blue), with increased cerebellar and DAN including DLPFC connectivity (red) comparing PD-MCI to no MCI sub-groups (early DR components 1-10) (P < 0.001).

In addition, significant fALFF differences existed between PD-MCI and no MCI sub-groups at conventional low frequency (LF) band of 0.01-0.08Hz (higher in the PD-MCI group with P = 0.005), with trends of higher slow-wave sub-bands of S5 (0.01-0.027 Hz; P = 0.127) and S4 (0.027-0.073 Hz; P = 0.211) (Figure 11). And small-worldness analysis based on fMRI connectivity data in two sub-groups found slightly decreased absolute global efficiency (Lamda, shortest path length) in PD with MCI sub-group (red dark line) compared to PD without MCI (blue light line), with the compensation of increased local relative efficiency (CCFS) in PD with MCI patients (Figure 12A). While the overall small-worldness factor (Sigma) was close, with slightly higher values at low-sparsity level comparing PD without MCI to PD-MCI sub-groups (Figure 12B).

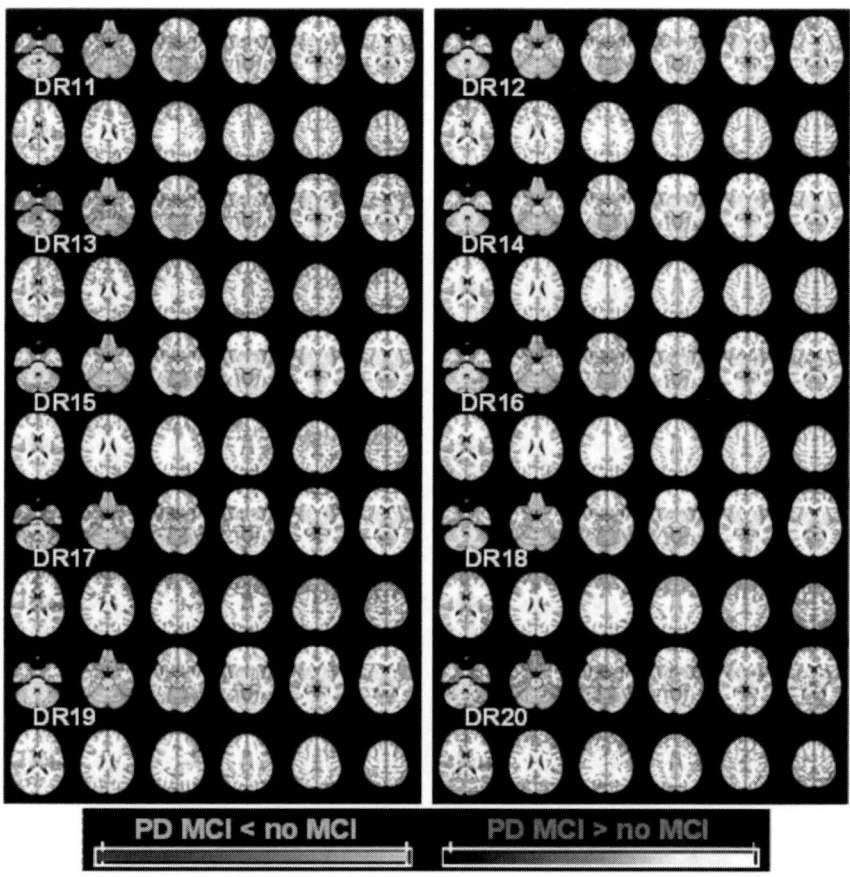

Figure 10. ICA-DR later components 11-20 comparing PD-MCI to no MCI sub-groups. Additional regions with connectivity deficits in anterior cingulate, motor cortex and basal ganglia were further observed in PD-MCI (P < 0.001).

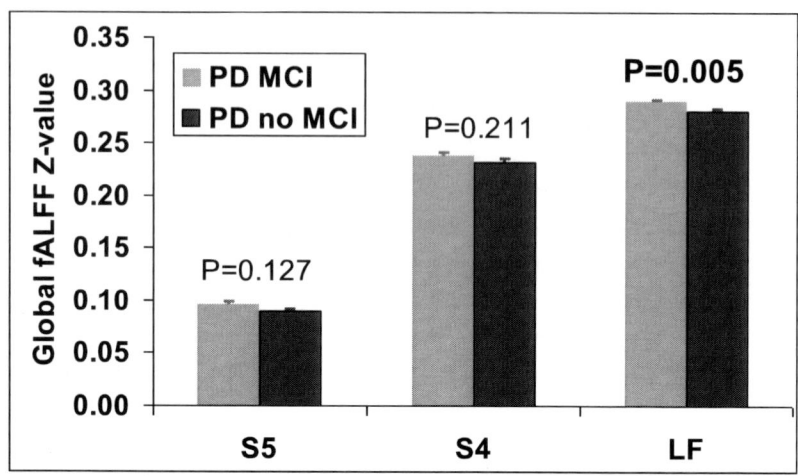

Figure 11. Significant fALFF differences between PD-MCI and no MCI sub-groups at conventional low frequency (LF) band of 0.01-0.08Hz (higher in the PD-MCI group; P = 0.005), with trends of higher slow-wave sub-bands of S5 (0.01-0.027 Hz; P = 0.127) and S4 (0.027-0.073 Hz; P = 0.211) in PD-MCI.

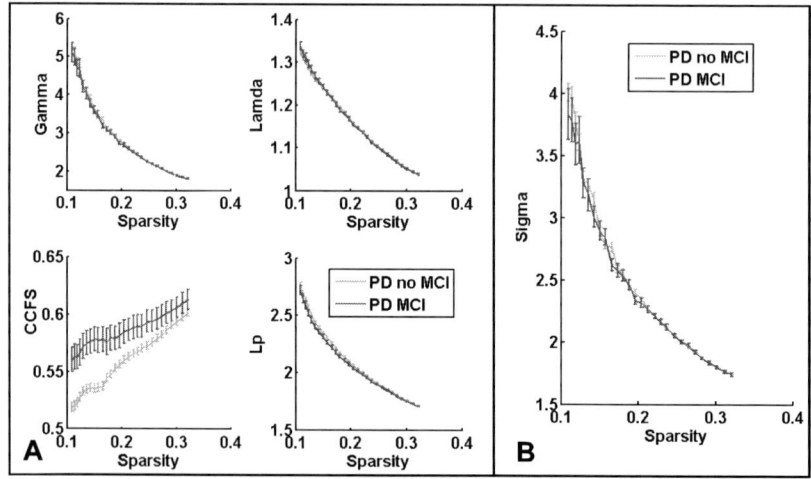

Figure 12. A: Small-worldness analysis based on fMRI connectivity data in two sub-groups showing slightly decreased absolute global efficiency (Lamda, shortest path length) in PD with MCI sub-group (red dark line) compared to PD without MCI (blue light line), and the compensation of increased local relative efficiency (CCFS) in PD with MCI patients. B: The overall small-worldness factor (Sigma) presented relatively higher values at low-sparsity level comparing PD without MCI to MCI sub-groups.

4. Discussion

In this work, expected volume atrophy in the hippocampus, especially significant and gradual volume reduction in the subfields DG and CA1 were observed from NC to EMCI and pAD progression. The typical global DMN network failure risk factor and several weighted sub-networks ratios were also increased in pAD compared to NC and EMCI groups. The multi-level intra- and inter- network connectivity using ICA-DR algorithm identified reduced inter- DMN-FPN, DMN-temporal cortex, FPN-temporal cortex and FPN-insular network coordination, together with lower intra-DMN (posterior cingulate) connectivity and intra-FPN nodes in MCI patients compared to controls. Typical functional compensation with increased inter- DMN/FPN and motor/supplementary motor networks were exhibited as well, in addition to the higher inter- DMN-basal ganglia and FPN-visual cortex correlations. The fcMRI results had been further identified with conventional seed-based RSFC such as decreased posterior cingulate and hippocampus fcMRI with increased connectivity in the hippocampus-DMN-supplementary motor regions [30]. These network connectivity changes were beyond the aging effects of lower DMN but higher DAN fcMRI, and might reflect the underlying neuropathological mechanism [32]. Furthermore, baseline amyloid and tau deposition predicted longitudinal tau change in multiple brain regions including the hippocampus and parietal region. Our previous results also reported longitudinal volume reductions in the hippocampal subfields of general EMCI (-2.5% per year) and pAD (-4.2% per year) groups; and were correlated with baseline amyloid and tau levels in multiple brain regions such as in the temporal cortex [31]. Baseline tau deposition and hippocampal volume correlated with longitudinal change of DMN fcMRI additionally. And strong correlations existed among multiple imaging metrics including DMN functional connectivity, hippocampal volume, tau deposition and structural connectivity; together with multiple cognitive tests such as memory and executive function scores [31, 33, 34].

The lower VMIIC (interhemispheric conductivity) in the hippocampus, anterior temporal and superior frontal were in agreement with the volume atrophy in these regions in PD-MCI compared to PD-no MCI sub-groups; together with both higher values in the visual cortex. The lower functional connectivity between hippocampus and IFG as well as between IFG and anterior temporal region had been reported, suggesting VMHC metric could also reflect multi-regional connectivity change [15]. The areas that presented no change of volume but higher VMHC in PD-MCI such as the orbitofrontal and inferior parietal regions might be recruited for functional compensation with preserved morphology, while lower conductivity in the substantia nigra swallow tail sign signature region indicated worse motor disorder in PD-MCI compared to no MCI sub-groups. Functional connectivity changes with ICA-DR algorithm identified typical network rerouting strategy such as decreased DMN/FPN, insular, anterior cingulate cortex, motor area and basal ganglia but increased DAN/cerebellum in early PD-MCI (MoCA score = 25) patients. These intra- and inter-network connectivity results, showing multi-domain deficits including memory, executive function, motor coordination and visual attention, were in line with previous findings using conventional RSFC methods [12-14]. Higher low-frequency functional activity together with lower global but higher local efficiencies in PD-MCI compared to no MCI sub-groups might be due to the over-recruitment of local neuronal resources in PD-MCI patients with systematic abnormalities.

Given the relatively high prevalence of PD-MCI over time, challenges still remain regarding standard diagnostic criterion and various domains of cognitive impairments in addition to the possible early prevention of progression to severe PDD [35]. Effective treatments including both pharmacological and non-pharmacological interventions are needed for PD-MCI patients; for instance, vitamin D for mood and olfactory function improvement in PD as well as brain stimulation for functional network modulation and normalization [36-38]. Olfactory impairments together with Aβ1-42 accumulation could lead to cognitive decline in early PD patients and progression to PD-MCI, with associated poor UPDRS motor scale and worse MMSE memory score [39, 40]. Higher education level and cognitive training for more brain reserve and less functional impairment risk, physical training such as aerobic exercise and proper nutrition for dementia onset delay in PD and better medication interaction are some recommended strategies for early comorbid disorder prevention and improvement in quality of life for patients [34, 41-43]. For both PD subgroup data cohorts, inclusion of more participants and integration with molecular imaging findings and multiomics will be some future work.

In conclusion, we had demonstrated hippocampal atrophy and disrupted brain networks including DMN and FPN in MCI and early AD population compared to NC with advanced imaging quantifications. MCI in PD, as a special case, also exhibited brain atrophy and interhemispheric dis-coordination in typical regions of substantia nigra, hippocampus, anterior temporal and superior frontal cortices compared to PD without MCI. Furthermore, decreased inter-network connectivity of DMN/FPN but increased DAN/cerebellum as compensation was identified in PD-MCI in addition to the decreased global efficiency together with increased local efficiency and low-frequency synchrony. Our results presented multi-level brain abnormalities including functional, morphological, micro-structural and molecular perspectives in general MCI at early stage as well as MCI in PD, and could provide solid imaging evidence for comorbid disease prevention and efficient treatment.

ACKNOWLEDGMENTS

Data collection and sharing for this project was funded by the Alzheimer's Disease Neuroimaging Initiative (ADNI) (National Institutes of Health Grant U01 AG024904) and DOD ADNI (Department of Defense award number W81XWH-12-2-0012). ADNI is funded by the National Institute on Aging, the National Institute of Biomedical Imaging and Bioengineering, and through generous contributions from the following: AbbVie, Alzheimer's Association; Alzheimer's Drug Discovery Foundation; Araclon Biotech; BioClinica, Inc.; Biogen; Bristol-Myers Squibb Company; CereSpir, Inc.; Cogstate; Eisai Inc.; Elan Pharmaceuticals, Inc.; Eli Lilly and Company; EuroImmun; F. Hoffmann-La Roche Ltd and its affiliated company Genentech, Inc.; Fujirebio; GE

Healthcare; IXICO Ltd.; Janssen Alzheimer Immunotherapy Research and Development, LLC.; Johnson and Johnson Pharmaceutical Research and Development LLC.; Lumosity; Lundbeck; Merck and Co., Inc.; Meso Scale Diagnostics, LLC.; NeuroRx Research; Neurotrack Technologies; Novartis Pharmaceuticals Corporation; Pfizer Inc.; Piramal Imaging; Servier; Takeda Pharmaceutical Company; and Transition Therapeutics. The Canadian Institutes of Health Research is providing funds to support ADNI clinical sites in Canada. Private sector contributions are facilitated by the Foundation for the National Institutes of Health (www.fnih.org). The grantee organization is the Northern California Institute for Research and Education, and the study is coordinated by the Alzheimer's Therapeutic Research Institute at the University of Southern California. ADNI data are disseminated by the Laboratory for NeuroImaging at the University of Southern California.

Data used in preparation of this article were obtained from the Alzheimer's Disease Neuroimaging Initiative (ADNI) database website (adni.loni.usc.edu). The author is one of the investigators of ADNI data cohort. The other investigators within the ADNI might contribute to the design and implementation of ADNI and/or provide data but did not participate in analysis or writing of this report.

REFERENCES

[1] Dong Y, Lee WY, Basri NA, Collinson SL, Merchant RA, Venketasubramanian N, Chen CL. The Montreal Cognitive Assessment is superior to the Mini-Mental State Examination in detecting patients at higher risk of dementia. *Int Psychogeriatr*. 2012 Nov;24(11):1749-55. doi: 10.1017/S1041610212001068. Epub 2012 Jun 12. PMID: 22687278.

[2] Hoops S, Nazem S, Siderowf AD, Duda JE, Xie SX, Stern MB, Weintraub D. Validity of the MoCA and MMSE in the detection of MCI and dementia in Parkinson disease. *Neurology*. 2009 Nov

24;73(21):1738-45. doi: 10.1212/WNL. 0b013e3181c34b47. PMID: 19933974; PMCID: PMC2788810.

[3] Tan JP, Li N, Gao J, Wang LN, Zhao YM, Yu BC, Du W, Zhang WJ, Cui LQ, Wang QS, Li JJ, Yang JS, Yu JM, Xia XN, Zhou PY. Optimal cutoff scores for dementia and mild cognitive impairment of the Montreal Cognitive Assessment among elderly and oldest-old Chinese population. *J Alzheimers Dis.* 2015;43(4):1403-12. doi: 10.3233/JAD-141278. PMID: 25147113.

[4] Ciesielska N, Sokołowski R, Mazur E, Podhorecka M, Polak-Szabela A, Kędziora-Kornatowska K. Is the Montreal Cognitive Assessment (MoCA) test better suited than the Mini-Mental State Examination (MMSE) in mild cognitive impairment (MCI) detection among people aged over 60? Meta-analysis. *Psychiatr Pol.* 2016 Oct 31;50(5):1039-1052. English, Polish. doi: 10.12740/PP/45368. PMID: 27992895.

[5] Saredakis D, Collins-Praino LE, Gutteridge DS, Stephan BCM, Keage HAD. Conversion to MCI and dementia in Parkinson's disease: a systematic review and meta-analysis. *Parkinsonism Relat Disord.* 2019 Aug;65:20-31. doi: 10.1016/j.parkreldis.2019.04.020. Epub 2019 May 7. PMID: 31109727.

[6] Hobson P, Meara J. Mild cognitive impairment in Parkinson's disease and its progression onto dementia: a 16-year outcome evaluation of the Denbighshire cohort. *Int J Geriatr Psychiatry.* 2015 Oct;30(10):1048-55. doi: 10.1002/gps.4261. Epub 2015 Feb 11. PMID: 25676160.

[7] Pfeiffer HC, Løkkegaard A, Zoetmulder M, Friberg L, Werdelin L. Cognitive impairment in early-stage non-demented Parkinson's disease patients. *Acta Neurol Scand.* 2014 May;129(5):307-18. doi: 10.1111/ane.12189. Epub 2013 Oct 11. PMID: 24117192.

[8] Martinez-Horta S, Kulisevsky J. Mild cognitive impairment in Parkinson's disease. *J Neural Transm (Vienna).* 2019 Jul;126(7):897-904. doi: 10.1007/s00702-019-02003-1. Epub 2019 Apr 8. PMID: 30963293.

[9] Hoogland J, van Wanrooij LL, Boel JA, Goldman JG, Stebbins GT, Dalrymple-Alford JC, Marras C, Adler CH, Junque C, Pedersen KF, Mollenhauer B, Zabetian CP, Eslinger PJ, Lewis SJG, Wu RM, Klein M, Rodriguez-Oroz MC, Cammisuli DM, Barone P, Biundo R, de Bie RMA, Schmand BA, Tröster AI, Burn DJ, Litvan I, Filoteo JV, Geurtsen GJ, Weintraub D; IPMDS Study Group "Validation of Mild Cognitive Impairment in Parkinson Disease." Detecting Mild Cognitive Deficits in Parkinson's Disease: Comparison of Neuropsychological Tests. *Mov Disord.* 2018 Nov;33(11):1750-1759. doi: 10.1002/mds.110. Epub 2018 Sep 14. PMID: 30216541; PMCID: PMC6261669.

[10] Goldman JG, Litvan I. Mild cognitive impairment in Parkinson's disease. *Minerva Med.* 2011 Dec;102(6):441-59. PMID: 22193376; PMCID: PMC3370887.

[11] Besser LM, Litvan I, Monsell SE, Mock C, Weintraub S, Zhou XH, Kukull W. Mild cognitive impairment in Parkinson's disease versus Alzheimer's disease. *Parkinsonism Relat Disord.* 2016 Jun;27:54-60. doi: 10.1016/j.parkreldis.2016.04.007. Epub 2016 Apr 9. PMID: 27089852; PMCID: PMC4887313.

[12] Gorges M, Müller HP, Lulé D; LANDSCAPE Consortium, Pinkhardt EH, Ludolph AC, Kassubek J. To rise and to fall: functional connectivity in cognitively normal and cognitively impaired patients with Parkinson's disease. *Neurobiol Aging.* 2015 Apr;36(4):1727-1735. doi: 10.1016/j.neurobiolaging.2014.12.026. Epub 2014 Dec 31. PMID: 25623332.

[13] Hou Y, Yuan X, Wei Q, Ou R, Yang J, Gong Q, Shang H. Primary disruption of the default mode network subsystems in drug-naïve Parkinson's disease with mild cognitive impairments. *Neuroradiology.* 2020 Jun;62(6):685-692. doi: 10.1007/s00234-020-02378-z. Epub 2020 Feb 17. PMID: 32064569.

[14] Shin NY, Shin YS, Lee PH, Yoon U, Han S, Kim DJ, Lee SK. Different Functional and Microstructural Changes Depending on Duration of Mild Cognitive Impairment in Parkinson Disease. *AJNR*

Am J Neuroradiol. 2016 May;37(5):897-903. doi: 10.3174/ajnr. A4626. Epub 2015 Dec 24. PMID: 26705323.

[15] Hou Y, Yang J, Luo C, Song W, Ou R, Liu W, Gong Q, Shang H. Dysfunction of the Default Mode Network in Drug-Naïve Parkinson's Disease with Mild Cognitive Impairments: A Resting-State fMRI Study. *Front Aging Neurosci.* 2016 Oct 26;8:247. doi: 10.3389/fnagi.2016.00247. PMID: 27833548; PMCID: PMC5080293.

[16] Zhou Y. *Joint Imaging Applications in General Neurodegenerative Disease: Parkinson's, Frontotemporal, Vascular Dementia and Autism.* Nova Science Publishers. 2021.

[17] Goldman JG, Bledsoe IO, Merkitch D, Dinh V, Bernard B, Stebbins GT. Corpus callosal atrophy and associations with cognitive impairment in Parkinson disease. *Neurology.* 2017 Mar 28;88(13):1265-1272. doi: 10.1212/WNL.0000000000003764. Epub 2017 Feb 24. PMID: 28235816; PMCID: PMC5373777.

[18] Bledsoe IO, Stebbins GT, Merkitch D, Goldman JG. White matter abnormalities in the corpus callosum with cognitive impairment in Parkinson disease. *Neurology.* 2018 Dec 11;91(24):e2244-e2255. doi: 10.1212/WNL.0000000000006646. Epub 2018 Nov 14. PMID: 30429273; PMCID: PMC6329325.

[19] Fornari LHT, da Silva Júnior N, Muratt Carpenedo C, Hilbig A, Rieder CRM. Striatal dopamine correlates to memory and attention in Parkinson's disease. *Am J Nucl Med Mol Imaging.* 2021 Feb 15;11(1):10-19. PMID: 33688451; PMCID: PMC7936250.

[20] Schrag A, Siddiqui UF, Anastasiou Z, Weintraub D, Schott JM. Clinical variables and biomarkers in prediction of cognitive impairment in patients with newly diagnosed Parkinson's disease: a cohort study. *Lancet Neurol.* 2017 Jan;16(1):66-75. doi: 10.1016/S1474-4422(16)30328-3. Epub 2016 Nov 18. PMID: 27866858; PMCID: PMC5377592.

[21] Keller SM, Gschwandtner U, Meyer A, Chaturvedi M, Roth V, Fuhr P. Cognitive decline in Parkinson's disease is associated with reduced complexity of EEG at baseline. *Brain Commun.* 2020 Nov

27;2(2):fcaa207. doi: 10.1093/braincomms/fcaa207. PMID: 33364601; PMCID: PMC7749793.

[22] Klassen BT, Hentz JG, Shill HA, Driver-Dunckley E, Evidente VG, Sabbagh MN, Adler CH, Caviness JN. Quantitative EEG as a predictive biomarker for Parkinson disease dementia. *Neurology*. 2011 Jul 12;77(2):118-24. doi: 10.1212/WNL.0b013e318224af8d. Epub 2011 Jun 1. PMID: 21633128; PMCID: PMC3140072.

[23] Cozac VV, Gschwandtner U, Hatz F, Hardmeier M, Rüegg S, Fuhr P. Quantitative EEG and Cognitive Decline in Parkinson's Disease. *Parkinsons Dis*. 2016;2016:9060649. doi: 10.1155/2016/9060649. Epub 2016 Apr 11. PMID: 27148466; PMCID: PMC4842380.

[24] Guner D, Tiftikcioglu BI, Tuncay N, Zorlu Y. Contribution of Quantitative EEG to the Diagnosis of Early Cognitive Impairment in Patients With Idiopathic Parkinson's Disease. *Clin EEG Neurosci*. 2017 Sep;48(5):348-354. doi: 10.1177/1550059416662412. Epub 2016 Aug 3. PMID: 27491643.

[25] Caviness JN, Hentz JG, Belden CM, Shill HA, Driver-Dunckley ED, Sabbagh MN, Powell JJ, Adler CH. Longitudinal EEG changes correlate with cognitive measure deterioration in Parkinson's disease. *J Parkinsons Dis*. 2015;5(1):117-24. doi: 10.3233/JPD-140480. PMID: 25420672.

[26] Kozak VV, Chaturvedi M, Gschwandtner U, Hatz F, Meyer A, Roth V, Fuhr P. EEG Slowing and Axial Motor Impairment Are Independent Predictors of Cognitive Worsening in a Three-Year Cohort of Patients With Parkinson's Disease. *Front Aging Neurosci*. 2020 Jun 18;12:171. doi: 10.3389/fnagi.2020.00171. PMID: 32625079; PMCID: PMC7314977.

[27] Cozac VV, Chaturvedi M, Hatz F, Meyer A, Fuhr P, Gschwandtner U. Increase of EEG Spectral Theta Power Indicates Higher Risk of the Development of Severe Cognitive Decline in Parkinson's Disease after 3 Years. *Front Aging Neurosci*. 2016 Nov 29;8:284. doi: 10.3389/fnagi.2016.00284. PMID: 27965571; PMCID: PMC5126063.

[28] Baik K, Kim SM, Jung JH, Lee YH, Chung SJ, Yoo HS, Ye BS, Lee PH, Sohn YH, Kang SW, Kang SY. Donepezil for mild cognitive impairment in Parkinson's disease. *Sci Rep.* 2021 Feb 26;11(1):4734. doi: 10.1038/s41598-021-84243-4. PMID: 33637811; PMCID: PMC7910590.

[29] Major ZZ, Vaida C, Major KA, Tucan P, Simori G, Banica A, Brusturean E, Burz A, Craciunas R, Ulinici I, Carbone G, Gherman B, Birlescu I, Pisla D. The Impact of Robotic Rehabilitation on the Motor System in Neurological Diseases. A Multimodal Neurophysiological Approach. *Int J Environ Res Public Health.* 2020 Sep 9;17(18):6557. doi: 10.3390/ijerph17186557. PMID: 32916890; PMCID: PMC7557539.

[30] Zhou Y. *Multiparametric Imaging in Neurodegenerative Disease.* Nova Science Publishers. 2019.

[31] Zhou Y. *Imaging and Multiomic Biomarker Applications: Advances in Early Alzheimer's Disease.* Nova Science Publishers. 2021.

[32] Zhou Y. *Functional Neuroimaging with Multiple Modalities: Principle, Device and Applications.* Nova Science Publishers. 2016.

[33] Zhou Y. *Mild Cognitive Impairment (MCI): Diagnosis, Prevalence and Quality of Life.* Nova Science Publishers. 2017 Chapter 1;1-46.

[34] Zhou Y. *Function and Metabolism at Aging: Longitudinal Neuroimaging Evaluations*, Nova Science Publishers. 2019.

[35] Litvan I, Aarsland D, Adler CH, Goldman JG, Kulisevsky J, Mollenhauer B, Rodriguez-Oroz MC, Tröster AI, Weintraub D. MDS Task Force on mild cognitive impairment in Parkinson's disease: critical review of PD-MCI. *Mov Disord.* 2011 Aug 15;26(10):1814-24. doi: 10.1002/mds.23823. Epub 2011 Jun 9. PMID: 21661055; PMCID: PMC3181006.

[36] Cammisuli DM, Cammisuli SM, Fusi J, Franzoni F, Pruneti C. Parkinson's Disease-Mild Cognitive Impairment (PD-MCI): A Useful Summary of Update Knowledge. *Front Aging Neurosci.* 2019 Nov 8;11:303. doi: 10.3389/fnagi.2019.00303. PMID: 31780918; PMCID: PMC6856711.

[37] Fullard ME, Duda JE. A Review of the Relationship Between Vitamin D and Parkinson Disease Symptoms. *Front Neurol.* 2020 May 27;11:454. doi: 10.3389/fneur.2020.00454. PMID: 32536905; PMCID: PMC7267215.

[38] Beheshti I, Ko JH. Modulating brain networks associated with cognitive deficits in Parkinson's disease. *Mol Med.* 2021 Mar 10;27(1):24. doi: 10.1186/s10020-021-00284-5. PMID: 33691622; PMCID: PMC7945662.

[39] Fullard ME, Tran B, Xie SX, Toledo JB, Scordia C, Linder C, Purri R, Weintraub D, Duda JE, Chahine LM, Morley JF. Olfactory impairment predicts cognitive decline in early Parkinson's disease. *Parkinsonism Relat Disord.* 2016 Apr;25:45-51. doi: 10.1016/j.parkreldis.2016.02.013. Epub 2016 Feb 19. PMID: 26923521; PMCID: PMC4825674.

[40] He R, Zhao Y, He Y, Zhou Y, Yang J, Zhou X, Zhu L, Zhou X, Liu Z, Xu Q, Sun Q, Tan J, Yan X, Tang B, Guo J. Olfactory Dysfunction Predicts Disease Progression in Parkinson's Disease: A Longitudinal Study. *Front Neurosci.* 2020 Dec 14;14:569777. doi: 10.3389/fnins.2020.569777. PMID: 33381006; PMCID: PMC7768001.

[41] Nicoletti A, Luca A, Baschi R, Cicero CE, Mostile G, Davì M, Pilati L, Restivo V, Zappia M, Monastero R. Incidence of Mild Cognitive Impairment and Dementia in Parkinson's Disease: The Parkinson's Disease Cognitive Impairment Study. *Front Aging Neurosci.* 2019 Feb 8;11:21. doi: 10.3389/fnagi.2019.00021. PMID: 30800065; PMCID: PMC6376919.

[42] Cammisuli DM, Bonuccelli U, Daniele S, Martini C, Fusi J, Franzoni F. Aerobic Exercise and Healthy Nutrition as Neuroprotective Agents for Brain Health in Patients with Parkinson's Disease: A Critical Review of the Literature. *Antioxidants (Basel).* 2020 May 5;9(5):380. doi: 10.3390/antiox9050380. PMID: 32380715; PMCID: PMC7278852.

[43] Aarsland D, Creese B, Politis M, Chaudhuri KR, Ffytche DH, Weintraub D, Ballard C. Cognitive decline in Parkinson disease. *Nat Rev Neurol.* 2017 Apr;13(4):217-231. doi: 10.1038/nrneurol.2017.27. Epub 2017 Mar 3. PMID: 28257128; PMCID: PMC5643027.

Chapter 2

CONVENTIONAL IMAGING BIOMARKERS OF ATYPICAL PARKINSON'S - CBS AND PSP

ABSTRACT

We had applied advanced MRI and PET neuroimaging techniques in various neurodegenerative diseases such as functional coordination and inter-network connectivity in typical PD and comorbid PD with MCI patients previously. The purposes of this study are to: 1. reveal the imaging differences in corticobasal degeneration (CBD) and progressive supranuclear palsy (PSP) compared to controls as well as the differences between these two sub-types; 2. investigate brain alterations with imaging data acquired under different conditions in two patient cohorts; and 3. perform comprehensive analysis such as tract-based structural connectivity and graph-theory based small-worldness as well as correlations among different neuroimaging metrics.

Typical brain atrophy, lower interhemispheric correlation, functional intra-/inter- dysconnectivity patterns and structural integrity deterioration were reported in CBS and PSP patients. Specifically, cerebellum, basal ganglia, most of subcortical regions and cortical motor/premotor and supplementary areas, insula, superior frontal cortex and parietal lobe demonstrated gray matter atrophy in CBS/CBD patients compared to normal controls (NC). PSP patients presented similar atrophy patterns as to CBS under resting state eyes closing (RS EC) condition, as well as during resting state physiologically unconscious (RS PH) situation. Comparing PSP to CBS under two conditions, gray matter atrophy in the cerebellum, visual cortex and striatum, but more gray matter density in the cortical parietal, scattered temporal, thalamus and superior frontal regions were present. VMHC patterns were similar in CBS patients compared to controls under two conditions; including lower interhemispheric correlations found in regions of motor, posterior parietal and insula, orbitofrontal, temporal lobe and visual cortices but higher VMHC values in the basal ganglia such as red nucleus, hippocampus, superior frontal and cerebellum. However in PSP patients, predominantly higher VMHC were present in most brain regions including frontal, occipital and parietal lobes under RS EC situation. In contrast, under the RS PH condition, similar VMHC pattern as of CBS comparing to controls was found in PSP, with a less degree of spatial spreading. Lower functional network connectivity in the superior frontal cortex, anterior cingulate cortex and anterior temporal lobe together with lower inter-network connectivity of visual-motor and frontal-cerebellum pathways were identified in CBS patients compared to NC. Lower frontoparietal network connectivity but higher visual-motor and orbitofrontal inter-network connectivity were observed comparing PSP to CBS patients under two resting state conditions. Also lower mean FA but higher axial/radial diffusivity values were found in PSP compared to CBS groups in several white matter tracts such as anterior thalamic radiation, uncinate fasciculus and cingulum connecting the hippocampus, with similar small-worldness characteristics between two patients population. Our comprehensive results also confirmed largely common imaging features of CBS and PSP; however, altered MRI patterns under different situations and between two patients population indicated distinct neuropathological disease mechanism.

Keywords: corticobasal degeneration, progressive supranuclear palsy, PET/MRI, dual regression, independent component analysis, voxel-mirrored homotopic correlation, small-worldness, efficiency, eyes opening, eyes closing, resting-state fMRI, physiologically unconscious, gray matter atrophy, voxel-based morphometry, diffusion tensor imaging, diffusivity, fractional anisotropy, tauopathy

1. INTRODUCTION

Corticobasal syndrome (CBS) is a rare Parkinson's symptom with abnormalities in both cortical region and basal ganglia. The neuropathology of corticobasal degeneration (CBD) includes neuronal loss, gliosis and tau deposition in the neocortex, basal ganglia and brain stem, with typical symptoms of limb apraxia, myoclonus, dystonia and alien limb [1]. Gray matter atrophies in the premotor and motor areas as well as insula in CBS patients had been reported; and other cortical areas involvement for each sub-type depending on distinct neuropathology such as frontotemporal loss for CBS- TAR DNA-binding protein (TDP) case but temporoparietal loss in comorbid CBS-Alzheimer's disease (AD) subtype [2]. As for clinical symptoms, CBS with alien limb syndrome had frontoparietal atrophy in addition to contralateral supplementary motor area (SMA) deficits with less involvement of frontotemporal and motor areas [3, 4]. Severe gray matter volume reduction in the subcortical putamen and thalamus in CBS compared to controls had been reported as well [5]. Furthermore, lower functional connectivity in the middle temporal gyrus and posterior insula in addition to the central operculum was observed comparing CBS to controls, together with higher connectivity in the anterior cingulum, caudate and superior frontal gyrus [5]. Also combination of gray matter density and network connectivity could classify CBS patients more accurately [6]. Finally, PET tau molecular imaging identified substantial tau plaques in the motor, corticospinal tract and basal ganglia region in CBS [7].

Progressive supranuclear palsy (PSP) is another atypical Parkinsonism, with supranuclear referring to the damage localized above the eye-moving centers (nuclei) in brain and palsy indicating disorder impairing eye movements [8]. Slightly different from CBS, gray matter atrophy was present in bilateral thalamus, anterior insular, midbrain and caudate in PSP patients compared to controls, with specific atrophy pattern in several brain and midbrain regions to differentiate from typical Parkinson's disease (PD) [9]. The tau deposition in PSP was related to the gray matter atrophy in frontal cortex and white matter deterioration in the motor tract as well as cortical hyper-connectivity [10]. Furthermore, abnormal small-worldness architecture was observed with higher local and global efficiencies but lower centrality configuration, possibly due to higher tau burden, disrupted cortico-subcortical and cortico-brainstem interactions such as damaged frontal and deep gray matter structure in PSP [11, 12].

Compared to the motor and cognitive problems in CBS, common clinical features of PSP patients included postural instability at onset, Parkinsonism, vertical supranuclear gaze palsy and possible speech and executive dysfunction [13]. CBS patients showed more supratentorial microglial activation and tau pathologies than PSP patients (both metrics were correlated in most areas), with less pathology in infratentorial structure [14]. Aside from distinct pathophysiology and clinical symptoms, some common imaging features were also found in both PSP and CBS patients; for instance, hypo-connectivity between visual and auditory network connectivity [15]. Differences existed as well including lower cerebellar-insular connectivity in PSP but higher salience-executive control network connectivity in CBS patients [15, 16]. In addition, prominent brain stem atrophy in PSP but more cortical and subcortical gray matter shrinkage in CBD patients was reported [17]. Longitudinally, greater rates of anisotropy reduction around the central sulci and diffusivity increase in superior fronto-occipital fasciculus were demonstrated in CBS compared to PSP patients [18].

We had applied advanced MRI and PET neuroimaging techniques in various neurodegenerative diseases such as functional coordination and inter-network connectivity in typical PD and comorbid PD with MCI patients previously [19, 20]. The purposes of this study are to: 1. reveal the imaging differences in two atypical PD - CBS/CBD and PSP compared to controls as well as the differences between these two sub-types of atypical PD; 2. investigate brain alterations with imaging data acquired under different conditions in two patient cohorts; and 3. perform comprehensive analysis in patients such as tract-based structural connectivity and graph-theory based small-worldness as well as correspondence among different neuroimaging metrics.

2. METHODS AND DATA

2.1. Participants and Data Acquisitions

MRI/PET Imaging data used in the preparation of this article were obtained from the ADNI database (http://ida.loni.usc.edu). The primary goal of ADNI has been to test whether serial MRI, positron emission tomography (PET), other biological markers, and clinical and neuropsychological assessment can be combined to measure the progression of mild cognitive impairment (MCI) and early Alzheimer's disease (AD). ADNI is the result of efforts of many co-investigators from a broad range of academic institutions and private corporations, and subjects have been recruited from over 50 sites across the United States and Canada. For up-to- date information, see www.adni-info.org.

Table 1. Demographic information of subjects for four imaging modalities in the 4RTNI data cohort, including three resting state (RS) conditions of fMRI and one DTI acquisition. The RS-fMRI comparisons included: 1-CBS patients vs. normal controls (NC; from the NIFD data cohort) at resting state using brain stem as motion restriction (RS BS) during image acquisition with eyes closed (EC) [20]; 2-CBS and PSP patients at resting state with eyes closing and staying awake (RS EC) for RS-fMRI data acquisition; and 3- CBS and PSP patients with eyes closing and remaining physiologically unconscious (RS PH) condition for RS-fMRI data acquisition. And finally for 4-DTI data, CBS and PSP groups were included with same diffusion weighting b-value = 1000 s/mm^2 used

Group	Age (Years)	Women N/%	Total N
1-EC NC (awake RS BS)	66.1 ± 1.0	9/100%	9
1-EC CBS (awake RS BS)	68.7 ± 0.8	3/50%	6
2-EC CBS (awake RS EC)	66.4 ± 1.7	4/57%	7
2-EC PSP (awake RS EC)	71.7 ± 2.7	7/78%	9
3-EC CBS (unconscious RS PH)	69.4 ± 1.9	8/89%	9
3-EC PSP (unconscious RS PH)	70.3 ± 2.3	4/44%	9
4-DTI CBS (b = 1000)	68.5 ± 1.0	22/65%	34
4-DTI PSP (b = 1000)	68.4 ± 1.3	25/66%	38

All the original imaging data used in this chapter were downloaded from the Frontotemporal Lobar Degeneration Neuroimaging initiative (FTLDNI or NIFD) center and the 4-Repeat Tauopathy Neuroimaging Initiative (4RTNI) program. The imaging protocols are similar for NIFD and 4RTNI that share the control database and the data are available from the ADNI laboratory of neuroimaging (LONI) center after approval.

Multiparametric MRI imaging data included structural MRI for voxel-based morphometry (VBM), diffusion tensor imaging (DTI) data and resting-state (RS)-fMRI data acquired at multiple conditions. The imaging data were processed with in-house software. The demographic information including age and gender participants of each modality and sub-type or category are listed in Table 1.

2.2. Imaging Parameters and Post-Processing

All MRI experiments were performed using the 3T MRI scanner with standardized imaging protocols. The 3D MPRAGE (TR/TI/TE = 2300/900/3.0 ms, flip angle = 9°, matrix size = 240 x 256 x 160, resolution = 1 x 1x 1 mm^3) was also obtained for reference image used in RS-fMRI connectivity/conductivity maps, as well as for structural voxel-based morphology (VBM) analysis. The MRI VBM results were obtained using the FMRIB Software Library (FSL, www.fmrib.ox.ac.uk/fsl) based on the 3D-MPRAGE structural data.

For the resting-state (RS)-fMRI data acquired with eyes closing under either relaxing or unconscious condition, a standard gradient-echo EPI sequence (TR/TE = 2000/27 msec, flip angle = 80°, number of volumes = 240, spatial resolution = 2.5 x 2.5 x 3.0 mm^3) was performed. For the resting-state (RS)-fMRI data acquired with brain stem for motion restriction for both CBS patients and controls, the MRI parameters for standard gradient-echo EPI sequence included TR/TE = 5150/31 msec, flip angle = 90°, number of volumes = 96 and isotropic spatial resolution = 2.2 x 2.2 x 2.2 mm^3. All RS-fMRI data were preprocessed with motion correction and outlier screening such as mean frame displacement (FD) < 0.6 mm to remove excessive motion.

The quantitative VBM, voxel-mirrored homotopic correlation (VMHC), fractional amplitude of low frequency fluctuation (fALFF) and seed-based resting-state functional connectivity (RSFC) as well as ICA-DR quantification were derived after processing and analyzing the fMRI and MPRAGE data acquired under three conditions as specified in Table 1, using the same methods as described in previous works [19, 20]. Systematic graph-theory based small-worldness analysis was also performed on the preprocessed functional connectivity with MRI (fcMRI) correlational data to investigate whole-brain functional network integration and specialization in these conditions.

DTI data was obtained with standard spin-echo EPI sequence (TR/TE = 8000/109 msec, flip angle = 90°, number of diffusion directions = 64, spatial resolution = 2.2 x 2.2 x 2.2 mm^3). DTI data were first pre-processed with the Diffusion Toolkit toolbox (http://tractvis.org) to obtain the fractional anisotropy (FA) and three diffusivity metrics such as axial diffusivity (AD), radial diffusivity (RD) and mean diffusivity (MD) values in original b0 space. For the FA/RD/AD/MD quantification, the FSL tract-based spatial statistics (TBSS) toolbox steps 1–2 (i.e. preprocessing, brain mask extraction with FA>0.1 and normalization) were used for registration of all participants' FA into the FSL 1-mm white matter skeleton template. The transformation of the individual FA data to the FSL Montreal Neurological Institute (MNI 1-mm isotropic resolution) common space were implemented with the nonlinear registration tool FNIRT based on a b-spline representation of the registration warp field. After normalization of FA map to the MNI space, tract-specific mean FA values were obtained in 20 main tracts from the well-defined probabilistic tract template (FSL/JHU ICBM atlas). These 20 tracts included bilateral anterior thalamic radiation, corticospinal tract, cingulum, cingulum of the hippocampus connection, inferior fronto-occipital fasciculus, inferior longitudinal fasciculus, superior longitudinal fasciculus, superior longitudinal fasciculus (temporal part), uncinate fasciculus and forceps major as well as forceps minor. Quantitative AD/RD/MD values were obtained by applying the same transformation from individual FA to template space and computed with tract-specific mean values [20]. Statistical comparisons between PSP and CBS groups were performed to the voxel-wise whole brain and 20 tract-based FA/AD/RD/MD data.

3. RESULTS

VBM results demonstrated gray matter atrophy in CBS and PSP groups ($P < 0.05$) compared to controls and the difference between two diseases (Figure 1). Regions in the brain stem, basal ganglia, cerebellum, subcortical regions such as hypothalamus, thalamus, ventral striatum, caudate and putamen, cortical superior frontal, posterior parietal, supplementary motor area, scattered occipital clusters, insular and hippocampus showed gray matter atrophy in CBS patients compared to controls, using brain stem as motion restriction during image acquisition at resting state (RS BS) (Figure 1A). On the other hand, higher gray matter density in scattered regions including the frontal pole, anterior temporal and lateral somatosensory cortex were found in CBS patients. Similar atrophy patterns with slightly less spatial spreading in PSP patients compared to NC under the resting state with either eyes closing (RS EC) and physiologically unconscious (RS PH) condition were demonstrated in Figure 1 B and C respectively ($P < 0.001$). Comparing PSP to CBS patients under RS EC condition, gray matter atrophy was identified in the superior fronto-parietal and motor regions; while clusters in the visual cortex such as lingual and calcarine, ventral striatum and cerebellum presented higher gray matter density (Figure 1D). Moreover, under regular RS PH situation, gray matter atrophy in the cuneus, thalamus and scattered temporo-parietal regions were found comparing PSP to CBS patients (Figure 1E); but regions with higher gray matter densities including lateral occipital cortex, cerebellum, frontal pole, subthalamic nucleus, sensorimotor and inferior parietal clusters existed in PSP.

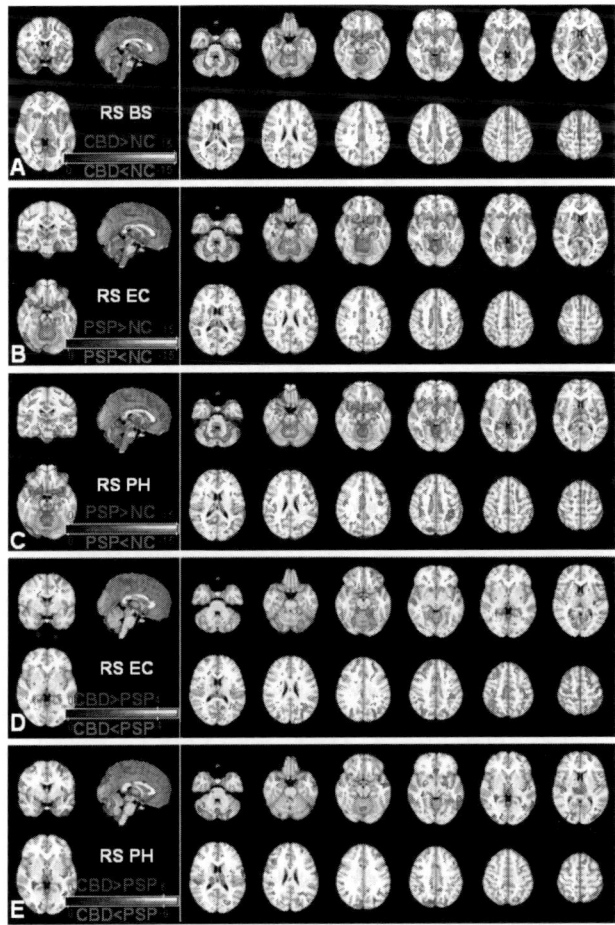

Figure 1. VBM results demonstrated gray matter atrophy in CBS and PSP and comparisons under different conditions ($P < 0.001$ for A-C and $P < 0.05$ for D-E). A: Regions in the brain stem, basal ganglia, cerebellum, subcortical regions such as hypothalamus, thalamus, ventral striatum, caudate and putamen, cortical superior frontal, posterior parietal, supplementary motor area, scattered occipital clusters, insular and hippocampus showed gray matter atrophy in CBS compared to NC under RS BS condition (blue color). On the other hand, higher gray matter densities in scattered regions including the frontal pole, anterior temporal and somatosensory cortex were found in CBS patients (red color). B and C showed similar atrophy patterns with slightly less spatial spreading in PSP patients compared to NC under the condition of RS EC and RS PH respectively ($P < 0.001$). D: At RS EC situation, gray matter atrophy existed in several clusters including visual cortex such as lingual and calcarine, ventral striatum and cerebellum comparing PSP to CBS patients (red color), while the superior frontal, parietal and motor/supplementary motor regions presented higher gray matter density in PSP (blue color). E: Under RS PH condition, gray matter atrophy was present in regions of lateral occipital cortex, cerebellum, frontal pole, subthalamic nucleus, sensorimotor cluster and inferior parietal lobe comparing PSP to CBS patients (red color), while the cuneus, thalamus and scattered temporo-parietal regions had higher gray matter densities in PSP patients (blue color).

VMHC differences between CBS and NC as well as between CBS and PSP under different situations were demonstrated in Figure 2 with P < 0.01. Comparing CBS patients to controls at RS BS situation, lower interhemispheric correlations were found in regions of motor area, posterior parietal and insula, orbitofrontal, temporal lobe and visual cortices (Figure 2A, panel A); with higher VMHC in the basal ganglia such as red nucleus, hippocampus, superior frontal and cerebellum. Quantitative information of brain clusters showing significant VMHC differences between CBS and NC under RS BS condition are listed in Table 2. Under RS EC condition, similar regions with lower VMHC including motor, posterior parietal and insula, temporal lobe and visual cortices but with less spatial distribution were identified in CBS patients compared to NC (Figure 2A, panel B with P < 0.01). However, higher VMHC in orbitofrontal, medial and superior frontal regions as well as cerebellum, midbrain and small visual clusters existed in CBS patients as well. Under the same RS EC condition, PSP patients presented mostly higher VMHC in several regions of frontal, occipital and parietal lobes, with lower VMHC in only small clusters of the anterior temporal lobe and superior frontal cortex compared to NC (Figure 2A, panel C). Also comparing PSP to CBS patients at RS EC situation, predominantly higher VMHC were found in the similar large brain regions as in Figure 2A panel A-C, including four lobes and somatosensory as well as medial frontal cortices (Figure 2A, panel D). On the other hand, slightly lower VMHC in small clusters of the anterior temporal region including the hippocampus, basal ganglia including red nucleus and substantia nigra, subthalamic nucleus, superior frontal area and cerebellum were present in PSP group as well.

Under the RS PH condition, lower VMHC in the motor area, subcortical peri-thalamic regions including thalamus, basal ganglia, subthalamic nucleus and insular, striatum including caudate, putamen and globus pallidum together with anterior temporal cortex and small orbitofrontal region were identified in CBS compared to NC (Figure 2B; panel A with P < 0.01). On the other hand, regions in the visual cortex, frontal pole, medial prefrontal cortex and cerebellum also presented higher interhemispheric correlation in CBS. PSP patients presented similar patterns of VMHC alterations as in CBS patients, but with a less degree of spatial spreading in several cortical regions (Figure 2B, panel B).

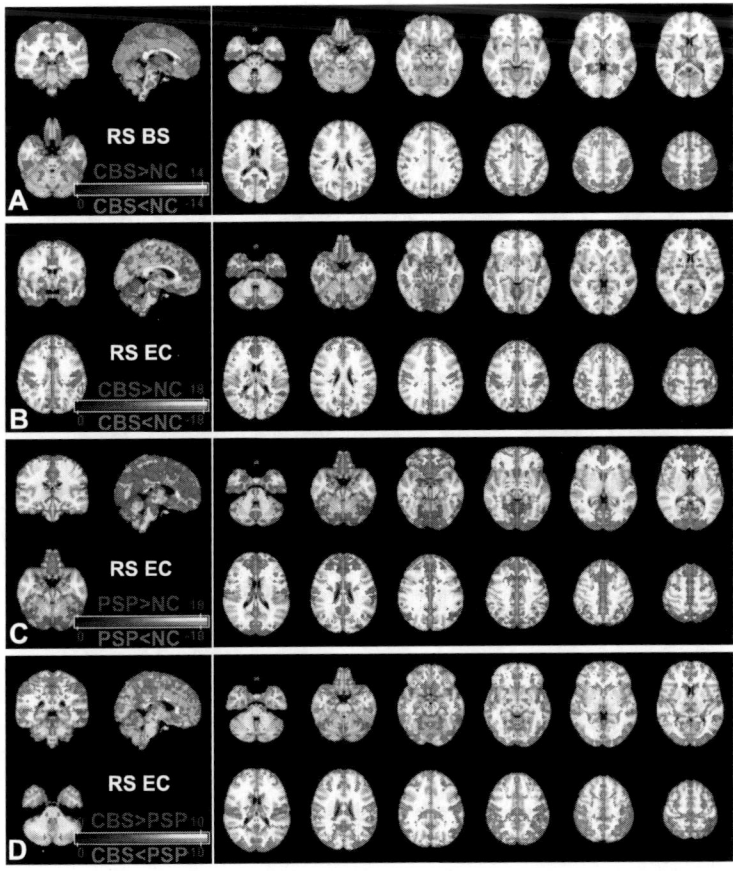

Figure 2A. VMHC differences between CBS and NC as well as between CBS and PSP under two different situations ($P < 0.01$). A: Comparing CBS patients to controls at RS BS condition, lower interhemispheric correlations in regions of motor, posterior parietal and insula, orbitofrontal, temporal lobe and visual cortices (blue color); but higher in the basal ganglia such as red nucleus and midline, hippocampus, superior frontal and cerebellum for CBS (red). B: Under RS EC situation, higher VMHC values were identified in larger areas in similar regions including motor, posterior parietal and insula, temporal lobe and visual cortices but with less spatial distribution were identified in CBS patients compared to NC (blue color, $P < 0.01$). However, higher VMHC in orbitofrontal, medial and superior frontal regions as well as cerebellum, midbrain and small visual clusters existed. C: Under the same RS EC condition, PSP patients presented mostly higher VMHC in regions of frontal, occipital and parietal lobes, with lower VMHC in only small clusters of the anterior temporal lobe and superior frontal region compared to NC. D: Comparing PSP to CBS patients at RS EC situation, higher VMHC in large areas as in A C; including four lobes and somatosensory as well as medial frontal cortices (blue); accompanied with lower VMHC in the anterior temporal region such as the hippocampus, basal ganglia including red nucleus and substantia nigra, subthalamic nucleus and small dorsolateral prefrontal cluster for PSP patients (red color).

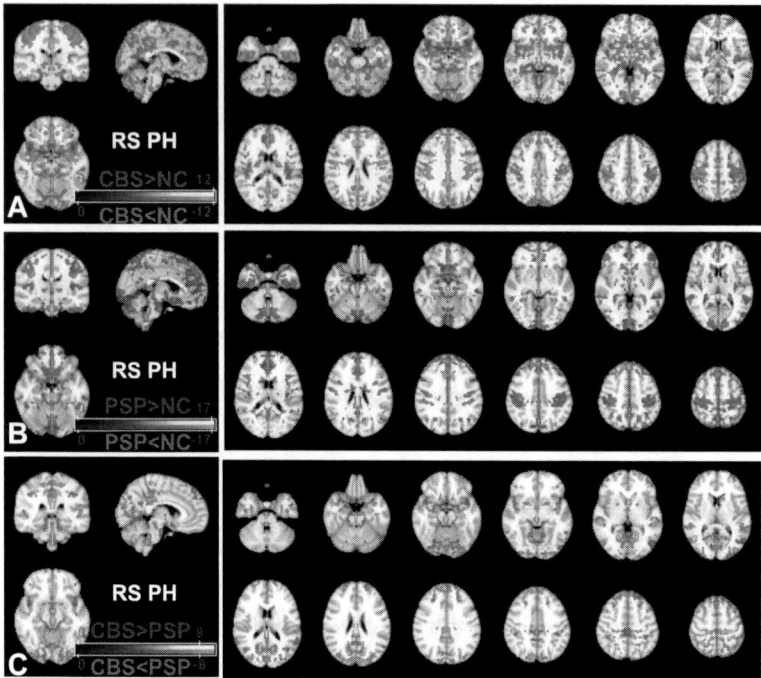

Figure 2B. A. Lower VMHC in the motor area, subcortical peri-thalamus regions including basal ganglia, thalamus, subthalamic nucleus and insular, striatum including caudate, putamen and globus pallidum together with anterior temporal cortex and small orbitofrontal region were observed in CBS compared to NC under the situation of RS PH (blue color, P < 0.01). On the other hand, regions in the visual cortex, frontal pole, medial prefrontal cortex and cerebellum also presented higher interhemispheric correlation in CBS (red). B. PSP patients showed similar patterns of VMHC alterations at the RS PH condition as in A-CBS patients, but with a less degree of spatial spreading in several cortical regions. However, basal ganglia midline, pons, hypothalamus, and amygdala in addition to the frontal and visual regions had higher interhemispheric correlation in PSP than NC (red color). C. The VMHC difference comparing PSP to CBS patients showed higher conductivity in midbrain and subcortical regions as specified in B, anterior temporal lobe and small superior frontal regions; but lower in visual, medial prefrontal and motor areas for PSP (all P < 0.01).

On the other hand, PSP had higher interhemispheric correlations in the basal ganglia midline, pons, hypothalamus, and amygdala in addition to the frontal and visual regions than NC. The VMHC difference comparing PSP to CBS patients showed higher VMHC in midbrain and subcortical regions as specified in panel B, anterior temporal lobe and small superior frontal region; but lower VMHC in visual, medial prefrontal and motor areas in PSP compared to CBS (Figure 2B, panel C and all with P < 0.01).

Figure 3 presented results of ICA-DR multi-component intra- and inter- network connectivity comparisons between CBS/CBD and NC. Ten representative inter- and intra- network patterns ($P < 0.01$) were selected: visual, thalamocortical, corticostriatal, cerebellum and basal ganglia networks; typical fronto-parietal network (FPN) and default mode network (DMN); motor, salience, frontal and temporal networks. Lower functional network connectivity in the superior frontal cortex, anterior cingulate cortex and anterior temporal lobe together with lower inter-network connectivity of visual-motor and frontal-cerebellum pathways were identified in CBS/CBD patients compared to NC (Figure 3). Higher network connectivity in the DLPFC, motor and supplementary motor areas, superior frontal and cerebellar regions existed, in addition to more inter-network connectivities of superior temporal, medial frontal-insular and visual-cerebellum circuits.

ICA-DR map comparisons between PSP and CBS/CBD patients under RS EC condition with $P < 0.01$ are illustrated in Figure 4. Lower FPN, DMN, insular, superior frontal region, temporoparietal and cerebellum connectivities were found in PSP compared to CBS patients. In contrast, higher inter-network connectivities in the visual-motor, thalamocortical, basal ganglia-sensorimotor, visual-orbitofrontal, motor-superior temporal pathways were found in PSP. Figure 5 showed ICA-DR map comparisons between PSP and CBS patients under RS PH situation ($P < 0.01$). Higher DMN, motor and supplementary motor areas, visual-motor and orbitofrontal connectivities were found in PSP patients compared to CBS (Figure 5 red color). Lower insular, frontal and parietal and anterior temporal regions existed as well.

Furthermore, lower FA values in PSP patients compared to CBS were found in most of distributed brain fibers using voxel-wise TBSS analysis. For instance, lower mean FA in several tracts including the anterior thalamic radiation, cingulum, inferior fronto-occipital fasciculus, minor forceps and inferior longitudinal fasciculus ($P < 0.05$) were identified in PSP compared to CBS patients as well as the cerebellar, basal ganglia and pons regions (Figure 6).

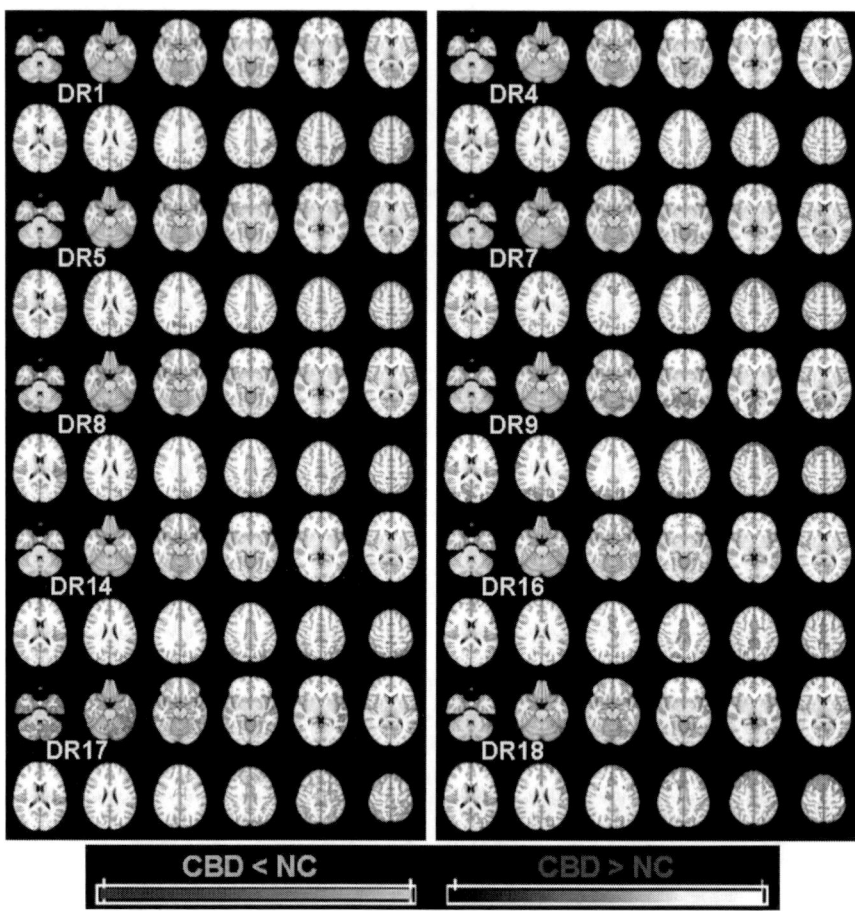

Figure 3. ICA-DR map comparisons between CBS/CBD and normal controls (NC) of representative DR components for ten different inter- and intra- network patterns (P < 0.01) at RS EC condition. DR1: visual network; DR4: thalamocortical network; DR5: corticostriatal network; DR7: cerebellum and basal ganglia network; DR8: fronto-parietal network (FPN); DR9: motor network; DR14: default mode network (DMN); DR16: salience network including insular, anterior cingulate and auditory cortex; DR17: frontal network including dorsolateral prefrontal cortex (DLPFC) and DR18: temporal network including inferior parietal lobe. Lower functional network connectivity in the superior frontal cortex, anterior cingulate cortex and anterior temporal lobe together with lower inter-network connectivity of visual-motor and frontal-cerebellum pathways were identified in CBS patients compared to NC (blue color). Higher inter-network connectivity in the DLPFC, motor and supplementary motor areas, motor-superior frontal and cerebellar regions existed in CBS, as well as higher superior temporal, medial frontal-insular and visual-cerebellum connectivities (red color).

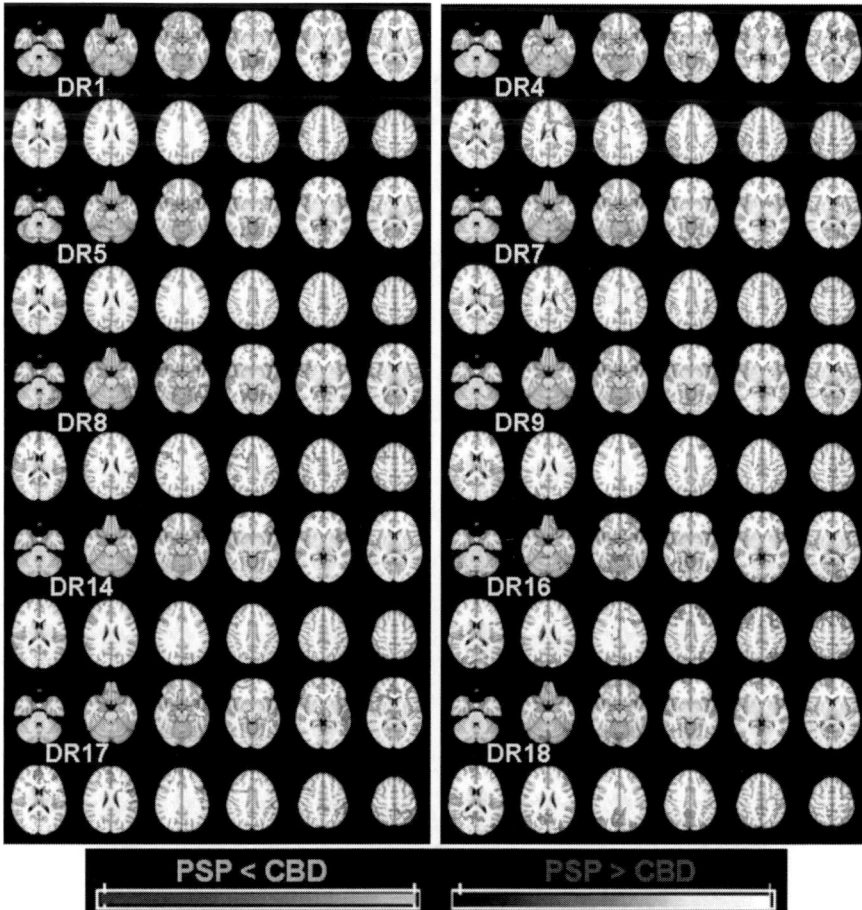

Figure 4. ICA-DR map comparisons between PSP and CBS/CBD patients under conventional resting-state eyes closed (RS EC) situation (P < 0.01). Lower FPN, insular, superior frontal region, DMN, temporoparietal and cerebellum connectivities were found in PSP compared to CBS patients (blue color). In contrast, higher inter-network connectivities in the visual-motor, thalamocortical, basal ganglia- sensorimotor, motor-superior temporal, visual-orbitofrontal pathways were found in PSP (red color).

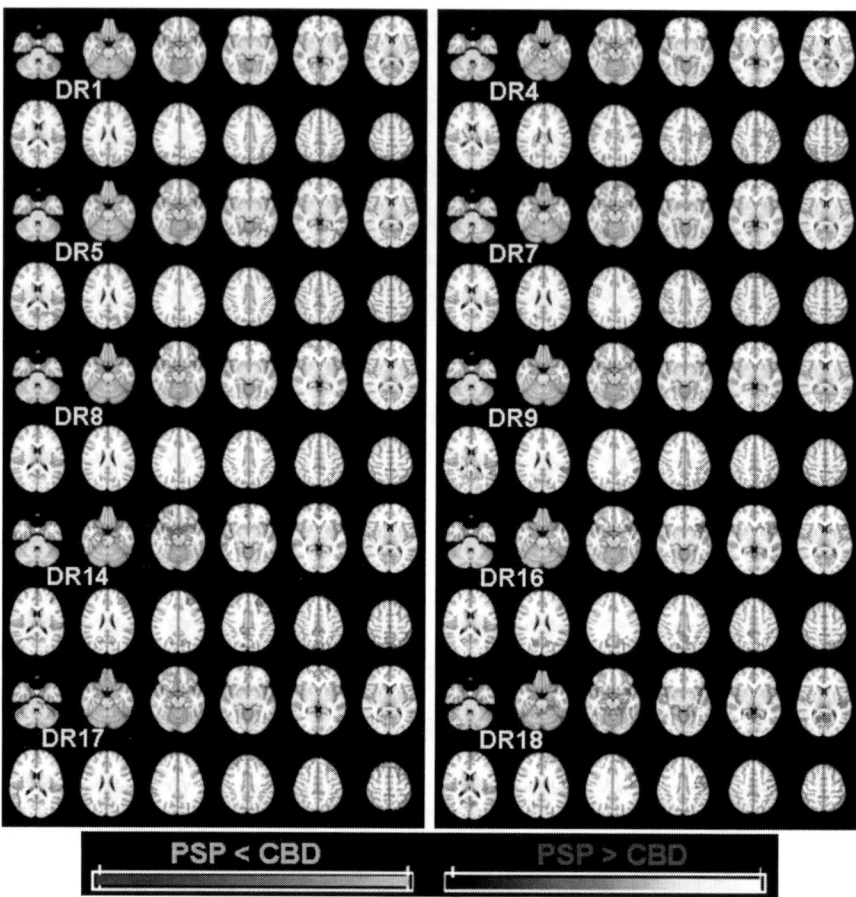

Figure 5. ICA-DR map comparisons between PSP and CBS/CBD patients under RS PH situation (P < 0.01). Higher DMN, motor and supplementary motor areas, visual-motor and orbitofrontal connectivities were found in PSP patients compared to CBS (red). Lower insular, frontal, parietal and anterior temporal regions existed in PSP patients as well (blue color).

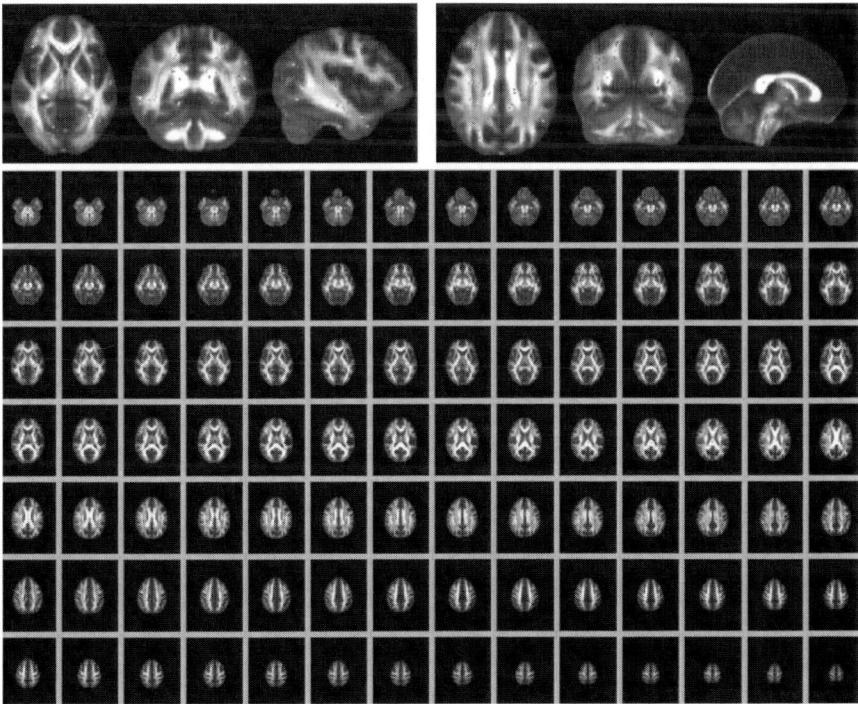

Figure 6. Lower FA values in PSP patients compared to CBS were found in majorities of brain regions using voxel-wise tract-based spatial statistics (TBSS) toolbox (hot color). For instance, lower FA in the anterior thalamic radiation, cingulum, inferior fronto-occipital fasciculus, minor forceps and inferior longitudinal fasciculus ($P < 0.05$) were identified for PSP group compared to CBS patients as well as in the cerebellar, basal ganglia and pons regions.

Figure 7 showed lower FA and higher diffusivity in PSP patients compared to CBS with the track-specific quantification. Specifically, lower mean FA in tracts of anterior thalamic radiation, right corticospinal tract, bilateral cingulum connecting the hippocampus, bilateral inferior fronto-occipital fasciculus, minor forceps, right inferior longitudinal fasciculus ($P < 0.05$) were identified in PSP compared to CBS patients (Figure 7; top two panels). Moreover, higher radial diffusivity (RD) in tracts of left anterior thalamic radiation, left cingulum connecting the hippocampus and bilateral uncinate fasciculus were found in PSP compared to CBS. And higher axial diffusivity (AD) in the similar tracts including left anterior thalamic radiation, bilateral uncinate fasciculus and additional superior longitudinal fasciculus (temporal part) were present in PSP patients (Figure 7; middle two panels). Finally, mean diffusivity (MD) values were also higher in left anterior thalamic radiation and bilateral uncinate fasciculus as well as left cingulum connecting the hippocampus in PSP compared to CBS (Figure 7; all with P < 0.05).

Table 2. Significant VMHC differences comparing CBS patients to controls with P < 0.01 using brain stem (BS) as motion restriction at resting state (RS) as in Figure 2A(A). Brain clusters on one side are listed due to the symmetrical interhemispheric computation

Brain Clusters	Cluster Size	P-value	MAX Z score	MAX X(vox)	MAX Y(vox)	MAX Z(vox)
A. Regions showing decreased VMHC in CBS patients compared to NC (P < 0.01)						
frontal pole	16532	0	12.5	42	90	59
temporal pole	1510	2.12E-11	7.58	21	66	14
cerebellum	1415	7.48E-11	8.4	42	23	14
temporal lobe	1253	6.85E-10	6.31	68	75	23
frontal lobe	618	1.31E-05	10.1	46	95	27
orbitofrontal cortex	295	0.00761	6.96	51	72	23
brain stem	289	0.00872	6.66	48	49	16
B. Regions showing increased VMHC in CBS patients compared to NC (P < 0.01)						
superior frontal cortex	1192	1.62E-09	8.64	40	84	64
middle brain	868	1.79E-07	8.35	44	66	19
brain stem	588	2.23E-05	14.5	44	43	0

Small-worldness based systematic analysis demonstrated lower relative local efficiency (Figure 8; Gamma) but higher absolute local efficiency (CCFS with large variation) in CBS patients compared to controls. Both relative and absolute global efficiencies (Lamda and Lp) were higher in CBS compared to NC. The scaled small-worldness factor (Sigma) was lower in CBS patients compared to NC, especially at low sparsity level (0.08-0.15). At the conventional RS EC situation, small-worldness characteristics were quite close in PSP and CBS patients (Figure 9). Under the RS PH situation, small-worldness characteristics were similar in PSP and CBS patients; except the absolute local efficiency (CCFS) was slightly lower in PSP patients compared to CBS (Figure 10).

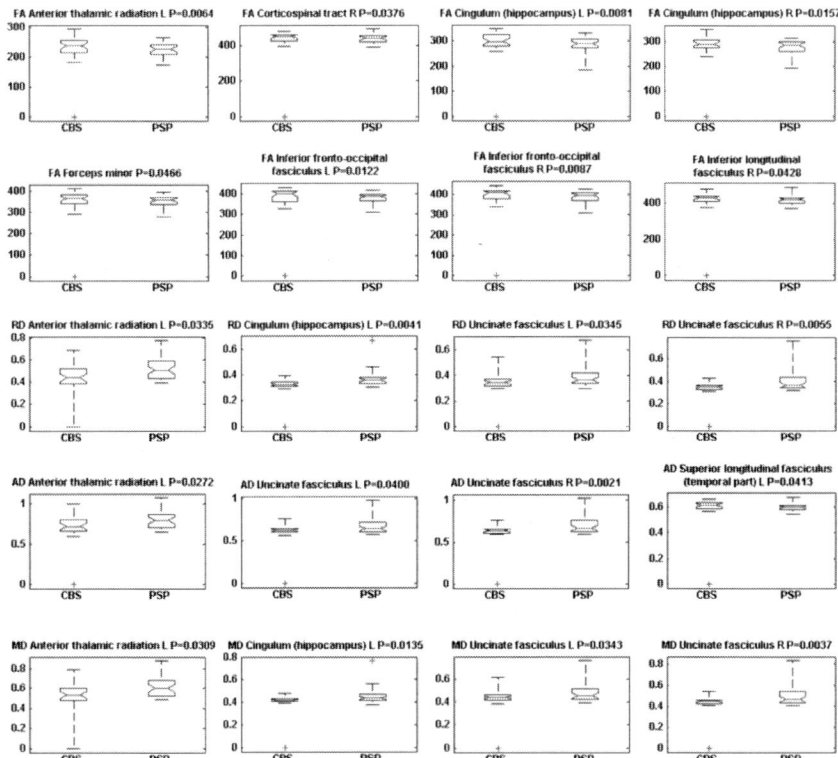

Figure 7. Lower FA and higher diffusivity in PSP patients compared to CBS were found in the track-based quantification. Specifically, lower mean FA in tracts of anterior thalamic radiation, right corticospinal tract, bilateral cingulum connecting the hippocampus, bilateral inferior fronto-occipital fasciculus, minor forceps, right inferior longitudinal fasciculus (P < 0.05) were identified in PSP compared to CBS patients (top two panels). Higher radial diffusivity (RD) in tracts of left anterior thalamic radiation, left cingulum connecting the hippocampus and bilateral uncinate fasciculus were found in PSP compared to CBS. Higher axial diffusivity (AD) was found in the similar tracts including left anterior thalamic radiation, bilateral uncinate fasciculus and additional superior longitudinal fasciculus (temporal part) in PSP patients. Finally mean diffusivity (MD) metric were higher in left anterior thalamic radiation and bilateral uncinate fasciculus as well as left cingulum connecting the hippocampus in PSP compared to CBS (all with P < 0.05).

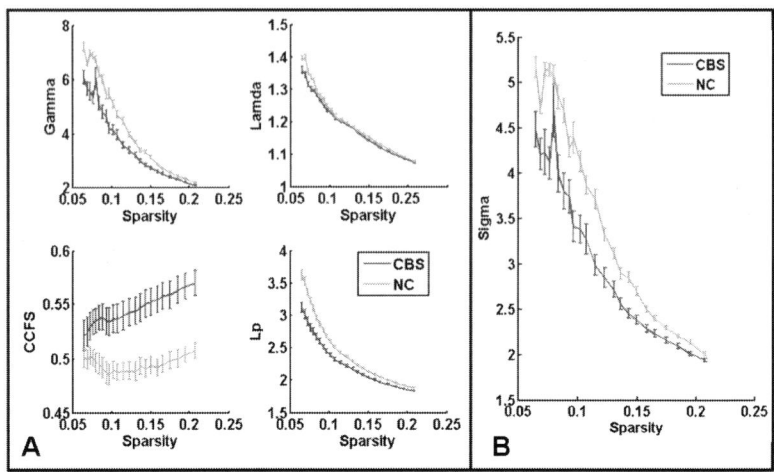

Figure 8. Small-worldness based systematic analysis demonstrated lower relative local efficiency (Gamma, red dark line) but higher absolute local efficiency (CCFS with large variation) in CBS patients compared to controls (blue light line) under RS EC condition. Both relative and absolute global efficiencies (Lamda and Lp) were higher (red dark line) in CBS compared to NC. B: The scaled small-worldness factor (Sigma) was lower in CBS patients compared to NC, especially at low sparsity level (0.08-0.15).

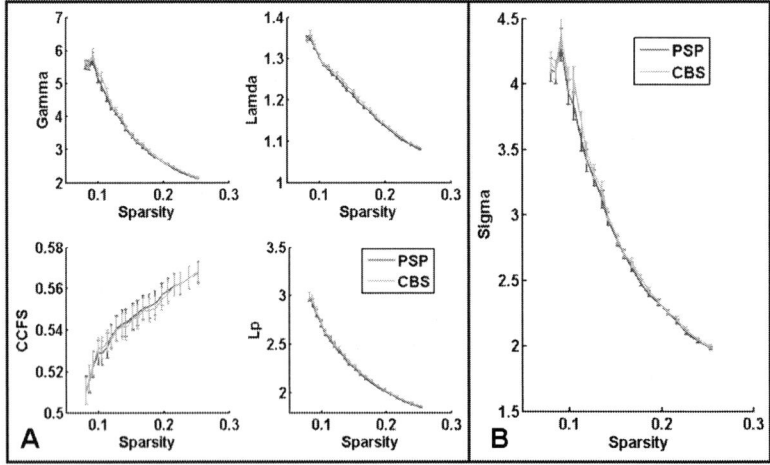

Figure 9. At the conventional resting state eyes closing (RS EC) situation, small-worldness characteristics were quite close in PSP and CBS patients.

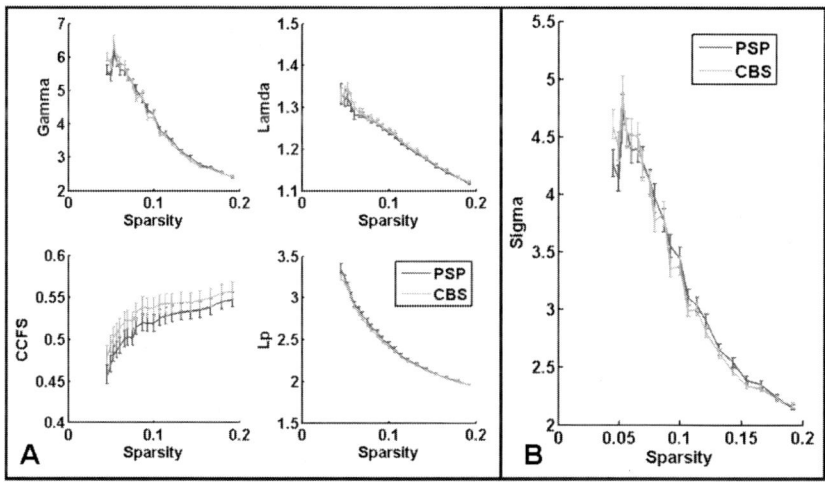

Figure 10. At the RS PH situation, small-worldness characteristics were almost identical in PSP and CBS patients; except the absolute local efficiency (CCFS) was slightly lower in PSP patients compared to CBS group.

4. DISCUSSION

4.1. Summary of Results

Our MRI results were consistent with previously published works, indicating multi-domain brain abnormalities in both CBS and PSP patients such as motor-related gray matter atrophies in CBS and visual/cerebellum deficits in PSP. Specifically, cerebellum, basal ganglia, most of subcortical regions and cortical motor/premotor areas, superior frontal and posterior parietal, insular, hippocampus, supplementary motor area, and scattered occipital clusters demonstrated gray matter atrophy in CBS patients compared to controls. PSP patients presented similar atrophy patterns as to CBS under both RS EC and PH situations. Comparing PSP to CBS under two conditions, gray matter atrophy in the cerebellum, visual cortex and striatum, but more gray matter density in the parietal, scattered temporal, thalamus and superior frontal regions were present in PSP.

VMHC patterns were similar in CBS patients compared to controls under two RS conditions; including lower interhemispheric correlations found in regions of motor, posterior parietal and insula, orbitofrontal, temporal lobe and visual cortices but higher VMHC in the basal ganglia such as red nucleus, hippocampus, superior frontal and cerebellum. And slightly higher VMHC values were found in the RS PH compared to RS EC conditions, mainly in the frontal, cingulum and visual regions. However in PSP patients, predominantly higher VMHC were present in most brain regions including frontal, occipital and parietal lobes under RS EC situation. In contrast, under RS PH situation, PSP showed similar VMHC pattern as in CBS comparing to controls, with a less degree of spatial spreading. Mostly higher VMHC values were found at RS EC condition comparing PSP to CBS. However, under RS PH condition, mostly lower VMHC in visual, medial prefrontal and motor areas and slightly higher in small midbrain and subcortical regions as well as anterior temporal lobe and small superior frontal region were present in PSP compared to CBS.

For the intra- and inter-network connectivity differences based on ICA-DR algorithm, lower functional network connectivity in the superior frontal cortex, anterior cingulate and temporal lobe together with lower inter-network connectivity of visual-motor and frontal-cerebellum pathways were identified in CBS patients compared to controls under RS EC condition. Higher inter-network connectivity in the DLPFC, motor and supplementary motor areas, motor-superior frontal and cerebellar regions existed, as well as higher superior temporal, medial frontal-insular and visual-cerebellum connectivities. Also under RS EC condition, comparing PSP to CBS patients, lower connectivity in the FPN, DMN and cerebellum connectivities were found in PSP but higher inter-network connectivities in the visual-motor, thalamocortical, basal ganglia-sensorimotor, motor-superior temporal and visual-orbitofrontal pathways existed. Moreover, under RS PH condition, lower connectivity in insular, frontal and parietal and anterior temporal regions but higher in DMN, motor and supplementary motor areas, visual-motor and orbitofrontal regions were observed comparing PSP to CBS patients.

For the DTI results, lower mean FA in tracts of anterior thalamic radiation, right corticospinal tract, bilateral cingulum connecting the hippocampus, bilateral inferior fronto-occipital fasciculus, minor forceps, right inferior longitudinal fasciculus ($P < 0.05$) were identified in PSP compared to CBS patients. Higher diffusivity with axial, radial and mean metrics in the similar tracts including anterior thalamic radiation and bilateral uncinate fasciculus were found in PSP compared to CBS. Graph theory based small-worldness analysis found lower relative local efficiency but higher global efficiency in CBS patients compared to controls. Both absolute local and global efficiencies were higher in CBS compared to NC but with lower small-worldness factor in patients, possibly due to the basal ganglia and cerebellum deficits with cortical function compensation in CBS. Small-worldness characteristics were similar in PSP and CBS patients under both RS EC and PH conditions, with slightly lower absolute local efficiency in PSP patients compared to CBS under RS PH situation.

4.2. Neuropathological Connection and Comparison with Previous Multimodal Findings Results

In both CBD and PSP patients, neurofibrillary tangles such as tauopathy and plaques are one of the causes, primarily the tau isomers with four repeats in the microtubule-binding domain (4R-tau) [13, 21]. TDP-43, RNA/DNA binding protein for metabolism and neurodegeneration mediation, together with copathology were present in 33% of CBD and 14% of PSP [21, 22]. Distinguishable brain patterns of tau propagation or spreading for each subtype indicated specific network involvement; for instance, predominantly subcortical pathology for PSP and mostly basal ganglia regions such as substantia nigra for CBD [23-25]. Investigation of the abnormal tau neuropathology and accurate *in vivo* quantification could help differentiation of CBS and PSP disorders [26, 27]. Neuropathological tau burden was also found to be associated with brain volume loss (atrophy quantified with MRI) in both CBS and PSP, but neurodegeneration score including neuronal loss was correlated with the superior-frontal functional connectivity metric only in CBD patients [28, 29]. In PSP patients, not only tauopathy but also cognitive impairment was connected with structural DTI alterations in corpus callosum and cingulum as well as gray matter atrophy [10, 30-32].

4.3. Diagnosis Improvement and Future Work

Morphological atrophy and structural dysconnectivity such as corpus callosum shrinkage in CBS and white matter integrity deterioration with lower FA and higher diffusivity in PSP were reported [33, 34]. Application of abnormal neuroimaging features could classify PSP and CBS patients from controls and predict clinical symptoms with high accuracies [35, 36]. Delineation of clinical phenotypes of CBS and PSP, as well as differentiation from other neurodegeneration types such as typical Parkinson's disease, frontotemporal dementia and Alzheimer's disease together with the imaging findings could improve diagnosis and prediction of underlying pathological mechanism [37, 38]. Specific tau isoforms could determine distinct neuropathological and clinical phenotypes for CBD and PSP, and might also help broaden the diagnosis criteria of each disease subtype [39, 40]. And finally, clinical trials targeting abnormal aggregation of tau accumulation with immunotherapy and genetic modification might offer some effective treatments [41]. Antipsychotics such as antidepressants for relieving behavioral symptoms and pharmacological agents for dementia and cognition improvement could be useful by minimizing adverse effects, optimizing patient management and improving quality of life [42, 43].

Taken together, typical brain atrophy, lower interhemispheric correlation, functional intra-/inter- dysconnectivity patterns and structural integrity deterioration were reported in both CBS and PSP patients at two representative conditions. Our results also confirmed largely common imaging features of CBS and PSP; however, altered MRI patterns of two special PD subtypes under different situations and between two patients population indicated distinct neuropathological disease mechanism.

REFERENCES

[1] Hassan A, Whitwell JL, Boeve BF, Jack CR Jr, Parisi JE, Dickson DW, Josephs KA. Symmetric corticobasal degeneration (S-CBS). *Parkinsonism Relat Disord.* 2010 Mar;16(3):208-14. doi: 10.1016/j.parkreldis.2009.11.013. Epub 2009 Dec 16. PMID: 20018548; PMCID: PMC2941264.

[2] Whitwell JL, Jack CR Jr, Boeve BF, Parisi JE, Ahlskog JE, Drubach DA, Senjem ML, Knopman DS, Petersen RC, Dickson DW, Josephs KA. Imaging correlates of pathology in corticobasal syndrome. *Neurology.* 2010 Nov 23;75(21):1879-87. doi: 10.1212/WNL.0b013e 3181feb2e8. PMID: 21098403; PMCID: PMC2995388.

[3] Albrecht F, Mueller K, Ballarini T, Lampe L, Diehl-Schmid J, Fassbender K, Fliessbach K, Jahn H, Jech R, Kassubek J, Kornhuber J, Landwehrmeyer B, Lauer M, Ludolph AC, Lyros E, Prudlo J, Schneider A, Synofzik M, Wiltfang J, Danek A, Otto M; FTLD-Consortium, Schroeter ML. Unraveling corticobasal syndrome and alien limb syndrome with structural brain imaging. *Cortex.* 2019 Aug;117:33-40. doi: 10.1016/j.cortex.2019.02.015. Epub 2019 Feb 25. PMID: 30927559.

[4] Rankin KP, Mayo MC, Seeley WW, Lee S, Rabinovici G, Gorno-Tempini ML, Boxer AL, Weiner MW, Trojanowski JQ, DeArmond SJ, Miller BL. Behavioral variant frontotemporal dementia with corticobasal degeneration pathology: phenotypic comparison to bvFTD with Pick's disease. *J Mol Neurosci.* 2011 Nov;45(3):594-608. doi: 10.1007/s12031-011-9615-2. Epub 2011 Sep 1. PMID: 21881831; PMCID: PMC3208125.

[5] Ballarini T, Albrecht F, Mueller K, Jech R, Diehl-Schmid J, Fliessbach K, Kassubek J, Lauer M, Fassbender K, Schneider A, Synofzik M, Wiltfang J; FTLD Consortium Germany; 4RTNI, Otto M, Schroeter ML. Disentangling brain functional network remodeling in corticobasal syndrome - A multimodal MRI study. *Neuroimage Clin.* 2020;25:102112. doi: 10.1016/j.nicl.2019.102112. Epub 2019 Dec 2. PMID: 31821953; PMCID: PMC6906725.

[6] Medaglia JD, Huang W, Segarra S, Olm C, Gee J, Grossman M, Ribeiro A, McMillan CT, Bassett DS. Brain network efficiency is influenced by the pathologic source of corticobasal syndrome. *Neurology.* 2017 Sep 26;89(13):1373-1381. doi: 10.1212/WNL. 0000000000004324. Epub 2017 Aug 4. PMID: 28779011; PMCID: PMC5649755.

[7] Smith R, Schöll M, Widner H, van Westen D, Svenningsson P, Hägerström D, Ohlsson T, Jögi J, Nilsson C, Hansson O. In vivo retention of 18F-AV-1451 in corticobasal syndrome. *Neurology.* 2017 Aug 22;89(8):845-853. doi: 10.1212/WNL.0000000000004264. Epub 2017 Jul 28. PMID: 28754841; PMCID: PMC5580862.

[8] Sobański M, Zacharzewska-Gondek A, Waliszewska-Prosół M, Sąsiadek MJ, Zimny A, Bladowska J. A Review of Neuroimaging in Rare Neurodegenerative Diseases. *Dement Geriatr Cogn Disord.* 2021 Jan 28:1-13. doi: 10.1159/000512543. Epub ahead of print. PMID: 33508841.

[9] Albrecht F, Bisenius S, Neumann J, Whitwell J, Schroeter ML. Atrophy in midbrain & cerebral/cerebellar pedunculi is characteristic for progressive supranuclear palsy - A double-validation whole-brain meta-analysis. *Neuroimage Clin.* 2019;22:101722. doi: 10.1016/j.nicl.2019.101722. Epub 2019 Feb 19. PMID: 30831462; PMCID: PMC6402426.

[10] Nicastro N, Rodriguez PV, Malpetti M, Bevan-Jones WR, Simon Jones P, Passamonti L, Aigbirhio FI, O'Brien JT, Rowe JB. 18F-AV1451 PET imaging and multimodal MRI changes in progressive supranuclear palsy. *J Neurol.* 2020 Feb;267(2):341-349. doi: 10.1007/s00415-019-09566-9. Epub 2019 Oct 22. PMID: 31641878; PMCID: PMC6989441.

[11] Cope TE, Rittman T, Borchert RJ, Jones PS, Vatansever D, Allinson K, Passamonti L, Vazquez Rodriguez P, Bevan-Jones WR, O'Brien JT, Rowe JB. Tau burden and the functional connectome in Alzheimer's disease and progressive supranuclear palsy. *Brain.* 2018 Feb 1;141(2):550-567. doi: 10.1093/brain/awx347. PMID: 29293892; PMCID: PMC5837359.

[12] Abos A, Segura B, Baggio HC, Campabadal A, Uribe C, Garrido A, Camara A, Muñoz E, Valldeoriola F, Marti MJ, Junque C, Compta Y. Disrupted structural connectivity of fronto-deep gray matter pathways in progressive supranuclear palsy. *Neuroimage Clin.* 2019;23:101899. doi: 10.1016/j.nicl.2019.101899. Epub 2019 Jun 15. PMID: 31229940; PMCID: PMC6593210.

[13] Litvan I, Grimes DA, Lang AE, Jankovic J, McKee A, Verny M, Jellinger K, Chaudhuri KR, Pearce RK. Clinical features differentiating patients with postmortem confirmed progressive supranuclear palsy and corticobasal degeneration. *J Neurol.* 1999 Sep;246 Suppl 2:II1-5. doi: 10.1007/BF03161075. PMID: 10525996.

[14] Ishizawa K, Dickson DW. Microglial activation parallels system degeneration in progressive supranuclear palsy and corticobasal degeneration. *J Neuropathol Exp Neurol.* 2001 Jun;60(6):647-57. doi: 10.1093/jnen/60.6.647. PMID: 11398841.

[15] Bharti K, Bologna M, Upadhyay N, Piattella MC, Suppa A, Petsas N, Giannì C, Tona F, Berardelli A, Pantano P. Abnormal Resting-State Functional Connectivity in Progressive Supranuclear Palsy and Corticobasal Syndrome. *Front Neurol.* 2017 Jun 6;8:248. doi: 10.3389/fneur.2017.00248. PMID: 28634465; PMCID: PMC5459910.

[16] Santos-Santos MA, Mandelli ML, Binney RJ, Ogar J, Wilson SM, Henry ML, Hubbard HI, Meese M, Attygalle S, Rosenberg L, Pakvasa M, Trojanowski JQ, Grinberg LT, Rosen H, Boxer AL, Miller BL, Seeley WW, Gorno-Tempini ML. Features of Patients With Nonfluent/Agrammatic Primary Progressive Aphasia With Underlying Progressive Supranuclear Palsy Pathology or Corticobasal Degeneration. *JAMA Neurol.* 2016 Jun 1;73(6):733-42. doi: 10.1001/jamaneurol.2016.0412. Erratum in: *JAMA Neurol.* 2016 Oct 1;73(10):1260. PMID: 27111692; PMCID: PMC4924620.

[17] Josephs KA, Whitwell JL, Dickson DW, Boeve BF, Knopman DS, Petersen RC, Parisi JE, Jack CR Jr. Voxel-based morphometry in autopsy proven PSP and CBS. *Neurobiol Aging.* 2008 Feb;29(2):280-

9. doi: 10.1016/j.neurobiolaging.2006.09.019. Epub 2006 Nov 13. PMID: 17097770; PMCID: PMC2702857.

[18] Boxer AL. Progression of Microstructural Degeneration in Progressive Supranuclear Palsy and Corticobasal Syndrome: A Longitudinal Diffusion Tensor Imaging Study. *PLoS One*. 2016 Jun 16;11(6):e0157218. doi: 10.1371/journal.pone.0157218. PMID: 27310132; PMCID: PMC4911077.

[19] Zhou Y. *Imaging and Multiomic Biomarker Applications: Advances in Early Alzheimer's Disease*. Nova Science Publishers. 2021.

[20] Zhou Y. *Joint Imaging Applications in General Neurodegenerative Disease: Parkinson's, Frontotemporal, Vascular Dementia and Autism*. Nova Science Publishers. 2021.

[21] Robinson JL, Yan N, Caswell C, Xie SX, Suh E, Van Deerlin VM, Gibbons G, Irwin DJ, Grossman M, Lee EB, Lee VM, Miller B, Trojanowski JQ. Primary Tau Pathology, Not Copathology, Correlates with Clinical Symptoms in PSP and CBS. *J Neuropathol Exp Neurol*. 2020 Mar 1;79(3):296-304. doi: 10.1093/jnen/nlz141. PMID: 31999351; PMCID: PMC7036659.

[22] Cho H, Choi JY, Hwang MS, Lee SH, Ryu YH, Lee MS, Lyoo CH. Subcortical 18 F-AV-1451 binding patterns in progressive supranuclear palsy. *Mov Disord*. 2017 Jan;32(1):134-140. doi: 10.1002/mds.26844. Epub 2016 Nov 3. PMID: 27813160.

[23] Dickson DW. Neuropathologic differentiation of progressive supranuclear palsy and corticobasal degeneration. *J Neurol*. 1999 Sep;246 Suppl 2:II6-15. doi: 10.1007/ BF03161076. PMID: 10525997.

[24] Brendel M, Barthel H, van Eimeren T, Marek K, Beyer L, Song M, Palleis C, Gehmeyr M, Fietzek U, Respondek G, Sauerbeck J, Nitschmann A, Zach C, Hammes J, Barbe MT, Onur O, Jessen F, Saur D, Schroeter ML, Rumpf JJ, Rullmann M, Schildan A, Patt M, Neumaier B, Barret O, Madonia J, Russell DS, Stephens A, Roeber S, Herms J, Bötzel K, Classen J, Bartenstein P, Villemagne V, Levin J, Höglinger GU, Drzezga A, Seibyl J, Sabri O. Assessment of 18F-PI-2620 as a Biomarker in Progressive Supranuclear Palsy. *JAMA*

Neurol. 2020 Nov 1;77(11):1408-1419. doi: 10.1001/jamaneurol. 2020.2526. Erratum in: *JAMA Neurol.* 2020 Nov 1;77(11):1453. PMID: 33165511; PMCID: PMC7341407.

[25] Smith R, Schain M, Nilsson C, Strandberg O, Olsson T, Hägerström D, Jögi J, Borroni E, Schöll M, Honer M, Hansson O. Increased basal ganglia binding of 18 F-AV-1451 in patients with progressive supranuclear palsy. *Mov Disord.* 2017 Jan;32(1):108-114. doi: 10.1002/mds.26813. Epub 2016 Oct 6. PMID: 27709757; PMCID: PMC6204612.

[26] Parmera JB, Rodriguez RD, Studart Neto A, Nitrini R, Brucki SMD. Corticobasal syndrome: A diagnostic conundrum. *Dement Neuropsychol.* 2016 Oct-Dec;10(4):267-275. doi: 10.1590/ s1980-5764-2016dn1004003. PMID: 29213468; PMCID: PMC5619264.

[27] Alquezar C, Felix JB, McCandlish E, Buckley BT, Caparros-Lefebvre D, Karch CM, Golbe LI, Kao AW. Heavy metals contaminating the environment of a progressive supranuclear palsy cluster induce tau accumulation and cell death in cultured neurons. *Sci Rep.* 2020 Jan 17;10(1): 569. doi: 10.1038/s41598-019-56930-w. PMID: 31953414; PMCID: PMC6969162.

[28] Spina S, Brown JA, Deng J, Gardner RC, Nana AL, Hwang JL, Gaus SE, Huang EJ, Kramer JH, Rosen HJ, Kornak J, Neuhaus J, Miller BL, Grinberg LT, Boxer AL, Seeley WW. Neuropathological correlates of structural and functional imaging biomarkers in 4-repeat tauopathies. *Brain.* 2019 Jul 1;142(7):2068-2081. doi: 10.1093/brain/ awz122. PMID: 31081015; PMCID: PMC6598736.

[29] Alster P, Madetko NK, Koziorowski DM, Królicki L, Budrewicz S, Friedman A. Accumulation of Tau Protein, Metabolism and Perfusion-Application and Efficacy of Positron Emission Tomography (PET) and Single Photon Emission Computed Tomography (SPECT) Imaging in the Examination of Progressive Supranuclear Palsy (PSP) and Corticobasal Syndrome (CBS). *Front Neurol.* 2019 Feb 14;10:101. doi: 10.3389/fneur.2019.00101. PMID: 30837933; PMCID: PMC6383629.

[30] Kovacs GG, Lukic MJ, Irwin DJ, Arzberger T, Respondek G, Lee EB, Coughlin D, Giese A, Grossman M, Kurz C, McMillan CT, Gelpi E, Compta Y, van Swieten JC, Laat LD, Troakes C, Al-Sarraj S, Robinson JL, Roeber S, Xie SX, Lee VM, Trojanowski JQ, Höglinger GU. Distribution patterns of tau pathology in progressive supranuclear palsy. *Acta Neuropathol.* 2020 Aug;140(2):99-119. doi: 10.1007/s00401-020-02158-2. Epub 2020 May 7. PMID: 32383020; PMCID: PMC7360645.

[31] Cui SS, Ling HW, Du JJ, Lin YQ, Pan J, Zhou HY, Wang G, Wang Y, Xiao Q, Liu J, Tan YY, Chen SD. Midbrain/pons area ratio and clinical features predict the prognosis of progressive Supranuclear palsy. *BMC Neurol.* 2020 Mar 30;20(1):114. doi: 10.1186/s12883-020-01692-6. PMID: 32228519; PMCID: PMC7106781.

[32] Spotorno N, Hall S, Irwin DJ, Rumetshofer T, Acosta-Cabronero J, Deik AF, Spindler MA, Lee EB, Trojanowski JQ, van Westen D, Nilsson M, Grossman M, Nestor PJ, McMillan CT, Hansson O. Diffusion Tensor MRI to Distinguish Progressive Supranuclear Palsy from α-Synucleinopathies. *Radiology.* 2019 Dec;293(3):646-653. doi: 10.1148/radiol.2019190406. Epub 2019 Oct 15. PMID: 31617796; PMCID: PMC6889922.

[33] Talai AS, Sedlacik J, Boelmans K, Forkert ND. Widespread diffusion changes differentiate Parkinson's disease and progressive supranuclear palsy. *Neuroimage Clin.* 2018;20:1037-1043. doi: 10.1016/j.nicl.2018.09.028. Epub 2018 Oct 4. PMID: 30342392; PMCID: PMC6197764.

[34] Kouri N, Murray ME, Hassan A, Rademakers R, Uitti RJ, Boeve BF, Graff-Radford NR, Wszolek ZK, Litvan I, Josephs KA, Dickson DW. Neuropathological features of corticobasal degeneration presenting as corticobasal syndrome or Richardson syndrome. *Brain.* 2011 Nov;134(Pt 11):3264-75. doi: 10.1093/brain/awr234. Epub 2011 Sep 20. PMID: 21933807; PMCID: PMC3212714.

[35] Bisenius S, Mueller K, Diehl-Schmid J, Fassbender K, Grimmer T, Jessen F, Kassubek J, Kornhuber J, Landwehrmeyer B, Ludolph A, Schneider A, Anderl-Straub S, Stuke K, Danek A, Otto M, Schroeter

ML; FTLDc study group. Predicting primary progressive aphasias with support vector machine approaches in structural MRI data. *Neuroimage Clin.* 2017 Feb 6;14:334-343. doi: 10.1016/j.nicl. 2017.02.003. PMID: 28229040; PMCID: PMC5310935.

[36] Quattrone A, Morelli M, Williams DR, Vescio B, Arabia G, Nigro S, Nicoletti G, Salsone M, Novellino F, Nisticò R, Pucci F, Chiriaco C, Pugliese P, Bosco D, Caracciolo M. MR parkinsonism index predicts vertical supranuclear gaze palsy in patients with PSP-parkinsonism. *Neurology.* 2016 Sep 20;87(12):1266-73. doi: 10.1212/WNL. 0000000000003125. Epub 2016 Aug 24. PMID: 27558375; PMCID: PMC5035983.

[37] Ling H, Macerollo A. Is it Useful to Classify PSP and CBS as Different Disorders? Yes. *Mov Disord Clin Pract.* 2018 Mar 6;5(2): 145-148. doi: 10.1002/mdc3.12581. PMID: 30363457; PMCID: PMC6174492.

[38] Cotelli M, Borroni B, Manenti R, Alberici A, Calabria M, Agosti C, Arévalo A, Ginex V, Ortelli P, Binetti G, Zanetti O, Padovani A, Cappa SF. Action and object naming in frontotemporal dementia, progressive supranuclear palsy, and corticobasal degeneration. *Neuropsychology.* 2006 Sep;20(5):558-65. doi: 10.1037/0894-4105. 20.5.558. PMID: 16938018.

[39] Sergeant N, Wattez A, Delacourte A. Neurofibrillary degeneration in progressive supranuclear palsy and corticobasal degeneration: tau pathologies with exclusively "exon 10" isoforms. *J Neurochem.* 1999 Mar;72(3):1243-9. doi: 10.1046/j.1471-4159.1999.0721243.x. PMID: 10037497.

[40] Armstrong MJ, Litvan I, Lang AE, Bak TH, Bhatia KP, Borroni B, Boxer AL, Dickson DW, Grossman M, Hallett M, Josephs KA, Kertesz A, Lee SE, Miller BL, Reich SG, Riley DE, Tolosa E, Tröster AI, Vidailhet M, Weiner WJ. Criteria for the diagnosis of corticobasal degeneration. *Neurology.* 2013 Jan 29;80(5):496-503. doi: 10.1212/WNL.0b013e31827f0fd1. PMID: 23359374; PMCID: PMC3590050.

[41] Coughlin DG, Litvan I. Progressive supranuclear palsy: Advances in diagnosis and management. *Parkinsonism Relat Disord.* 2020 Apr;73:105-116. doi: 10.1016/j.parkreldis.2020.04.014. Epub 2020 May 25. PMID: 32487421; PMCID: PMC7462164.

[42] Lamb R, Rohrer JD, Lees AJ, Morris HR. Progressive Supranuclear Palsy and Corticobasal Degeneration: Pathophysiology and Treatment Options. *Curr Treat Options Neurol.* 2016 Sep;18(9):42. doi: 10.1007/s11940-016-0422-5. PMID: 27526039; PMCID: PMC4985534.

[43] Kompoliti K, Goetz CG, Boeve BF, Maraganore DM, Ahlskog JE, Marsden CD, Bhatia KP, Greene PE, Przedborski S, Seal EC, Burns RS, Hauser RA, Gauger LL, Factor SA, Molho ES, Riley DE. Clinical presentation and pharmacological therapy in corticobasal degeneration. *Arch Neurol.* 1998 Jul;55(7):957-61. doi: 10.1001/archneur.55.7.957. PMID: 9678313.

Chapter 3

NOVEL IMAGING BIOMARKERS IN CBS/PSP AND ASYMPTOMATIC/ SYMPTOMATIC ALZHEIMER'S

ABSTRACT

There have been numerous studies investigating improvement of pattern recognition and revealing the underlying temporal dynamics in large-scale networks with more adaptive and better-characterized methods such as dynamic functional network connectivity (dFNC) algorithm. The specific objectives of this chapter are to: 1. explore further dFNC differences between two atypical PD groups -CBS and PSP under two resting state (RS) conditions, in addition to conventional imaging findings in Chapter 2; and 2. introduce as well as analyze some other novel imaging data such as cerebral blood flow with arterial spin labeling technique and PET/MRI correlation in early and asymptomatic Alzheimer's disease (AD).

Our results demonstrated dFNC differences between CBS and PSP under both resting state eyes closing (RS EC) and physiological unconsciousness (RS PH) conditions and confirmed the lower temporal dynamics in PSP compared to CBS patients. For instance, under RS EC condition, both lower salience network (SN) and central executive network (CEN) dynamic transition with dFNC method and hypo-network modulation with ICA-DR algorithm were in agreement in PSP compared to CBS participants. Also under RS PH condition, lower SN dFNC in PSP compared to CBS was similar to the ICA-DR inter-network modulation result as well as RS EC dFNC finding. Disruption of SN dynamics under both RS conditions was probably related to the disinhibition function that was common to both PD subtypes and state-shifting role of SN. Observations of lower interhemispheric conductivity, white matter micro-structural connectivity deterioration, inter-network dis-coordination and less temporal dynamics were consistent, indicating possible spatiotemporal communication and pathway distortion at different degrees in two patient cohorts. Moreover, we found significantly lower cerebral blood flow (CBF) values measured with MRI arterial spin labeling (ASL) technique in MCI/AD compared to controls ($P < 0.05$) for most ROIs, with a lower trend in AD compared to MCI. Strong correlations between CBF and memory composite score were present more in controls, less in MCI and AD patients; and CBF in a few regions correlated with language composite score only in AD. Also, significant associations between amyloid deposition in the anterior cingulate/orbito-medial prefrontal regions and MRI temporoparietal volume were identified in asymptomatic Aβ+ carriers. The combination of these novel imaging metrics such as dFNC and ASL-CBF together with conventional imaging quantifications could improve disease detection accuracy and validate the multiparametric metrics with better interpretation.

Keywords: corticobasal degeneration, progressive supranuclear palsy, dynamic functional network connectivity, temporal dynamics, state, connectogram, default mode network, frontoparietal network, salience network, motor network, visual network, central executive network, dwell time, frequency, occupancy, eyes opening, eyes closing, resting-state fMRI, physiologically unconscious, Alzheimer's disease, cerebral blood flow, arterial spin labeling, PET/MRI, mild cognitive impairment, volumetry, composite score, phenotypic harmonic score, amyloid, correlational test

1. INTRODUCTION

In addition to the conventional statistical correlation map computed between time series of seed and targeted voxel/regions, dynamic functional network connectivity (dFNC) had recently been proposed to cluster brain networks based on segmented and shifted characteristic time courses [1, 2]. Temporal variation and associated spatial map of all dFNC matrices could be derived using the multivariate decomposition method such as independent component analysis (ICA) and Markov modeling to obtain the most essential and informative source. State is defined as a statistical spatial pattern (projected correlation matrix) extracted from sampled dynamic windows that all participants most likely return or stay during the time course of the experiment [3]. With advanced modeling and clustering methods, dFNC had been applied to study the functional coordination and flexibility among different networks (inter-network connectivities) for better understanding of behavioral-related shifts such as vigilance/arousal and brain cognitive adaption processes [2, 4-5]. Similar to the ICA-based dual-regression (ICA-DR) modeling of multiple networks, dFNC could simplify and reveal the transit interactions between large-scale networks in comparison to the conventional static network analysis [6, 7].

Several issues raised regarding the dynamic temporal correlation computation and analysis framework such as window size selection and automatic clustering improvement [8]. The sliding-window size for dynamic correlation should not be too small to generate unnecessary transitions and not too large to filter out valuable variations, and window-size of 30–60 seconds was recommended for robust estimation of the dynamic fluctuations in resting-state (RS) dFNC [9]. Also detection power of dynamic functional connectivity could be increased by averaging across sessions and subjects [10]. The statistical validity, physiological origin and cognitive relevance are also some ongoing topics that could advance interpretation and generalization of this relatively new method [11]. Test-retest reliability for dynamic correlation and state statistics were assessed with confirmed outperformance, especially the dynamic correlation variance that was more informative [12]. Moreover, a decentralized dFNC provided comparable performance as to specific individual components, and could facilitate collaboration and data sharing among neuroimaging centers [13].

As to the physiologic origin, dFNC and dynamic fractional amplitude of low frequency fluctuation (fALFF) presented concurrent patterns and both were significantly related to cognitive tests, indicating dFNC might be close to the intrinsic neuronal activity [14]. At both eyes closing and opening conditions, state of higher thalamocortical anticorrelation was linked to higher EEG power spectrum of delta and theta bands but lower in alpha band and occurred more frequently in eyes closing situation, suggesting possible vigilance state and shift existence via dFNC analysis [15]. Furthermore, simultaneous fMRI and EEG data demonstrated the correspondence of dFNC states of fMRI signals to non-rapid eye movement sleep stages and slow-wave activity consistently, confirming the electrophysiological source of quantitative dFNC sensitivities and state-dependent fluctuations [16]. Another study had also validated variability of dFNC together with static default mode network (DMN) functional connectivity decrement during deep sleep [17].

Disease classification with fMRI data using dFNC algorithm had achieved remarkable accuracy for distinguishing different neurological disorders and neuropsychological diseases such as Parkinson's disease (PD), schizophrenia, traumatic brain injury (TBI), Alzheimer's disease (AD) and mild cognitive impairment (MCI) [18, 19]. For instance, abnormal brain network dynamics in PD patients compared to controls had been reported with a shift of dwell time between states and greater intra-network variability such as between cerebellum and auditory sub-networks [20, 21]. Also compared to PD without MCI, PD with MCI patients showed dFNC deteriorations with mostly lower inter- somatomotor and central executive network dynamic connectivity; however, higher inter-network connectivity and hyper-synchronization between basal ganglia and cortical motor circuits were often present in PD patients at baseline and longitudinal follow-ups [22-24]. In TBI patients, dFNC states with higher inter- cerebellum and sensorimotor dynamic values were selected as the imaging feature that had achieved 92% accuracy for patient classification. Also the number of group-ICA components, size of sliding-window together with spike correction preprocessing were found to be critical in optimizing classification performance for TBI [25, 26]. In mild AD, dFNC was reduced between visual and sensorimotor networks with less state time compared to controls, and certain dynamic features such as higher dwell time were associated with language and cognitive scores in AD [27-28].

There have been numerous studies investigating improvement of pattern recognition and revealing the underlying temporal dynamics in large-scale networks with more adaptive and better-characterized methods such as dFNC algorithm [29-31]. The applications of these relatively new techniques in neuroscience and various diseases could help interpret brain organization and optimal integration at normal states (similar to conventional methods), as well as confirm neuropathological findings and possibly provide objective and complementary information and state-based evidence [32-35]. The purpose of this chapter is to explore further dFNC differences between two atypical PD groups - CBS and PSP under two resting state conditions, to complement and validate the conventional imaging findings in previous chapter. Some other novel imaging findings in AD are also demonstrated.

2. METHODS AND DATA

2.1. Dynamic Functional Connectivity Network (dFNC)

Group ICA of fMRI Toolbox (Gift) developed at the Translational Research in Neuroimaging & Data Science (TReNDS, www.trendscenter.org/software/gift) center was used to derive the relatively new dFNC and connectogram results [1, 2]. The dynamic correlation matrix between well-known networks was estimated by means of the sliding-window approach that divided total time points for each participant into smaller segments, with close to optimal length of 22 TRs (= 44 sec) in our datasets. And independent vector analysis (IVA) with multivariate Gaussian and Laplace component vectors (IVA-GL) algorithm was applied to the smaller segments to derive the dynamic correlation matrices by obtaining the best performance with maximal mutual information and optimal complexity. Also Markov chain modeling was chosen to examine the connectivity dynamics with each k-means cluster representing a state, and the number of clusters could be determined by the elbow criterion to maximize the within-cluster to between-cluster dissimilarity [36-38].

Briefly four steps were involved in the computation of dFNC based on the algorithms aforementioned (Figure 1). Firstly, temporal ICA decomposition was used to the preprocessed functional data of each group to generate the spatial maps, time courses and power spectrum of all independent components. RS-fMRI Preprocessing steps involved primarily realignment, spatial smoothing, band pass temporal filtering of 0.01-0.1Hz, detrending, removal of nuisance signals such as motion parameters and global signal as well as transformation to the Montreal neurologic institute (MNI) standard space [6, 7]. Then, based on these ICA source components, several typical and important functional networks were chosen for connectogram construction, such as six dFNCs used in this work including default mode network (DMN), frontoparietal network (FPN), salience network (SN), motor network (MN), visual network (VN) and central executive network (CEN) or EN. Next, K-means clustering method and Markov modeling was applied to classify the temporal vectors (windows) into six clusters or six states based on multiple dynamic correlation matrices. Finally, statistical quantifications such as connectogram occurrence, frequency and mean dwell time were derived to characterize dynamics of these intrinsic temporal states [39-42].

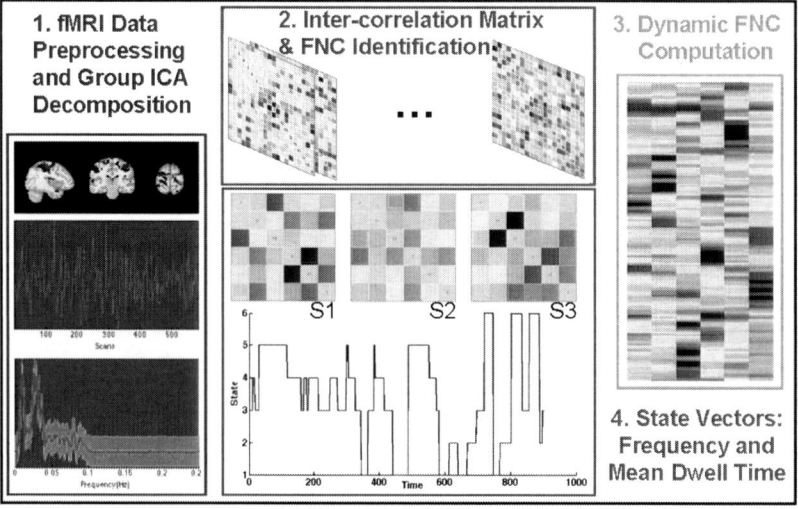

Figure 1. Outline of the dynamic functional network connectivity (dFNC) computation procedure steps used in Gift software [1, 2].

In addition to the typical imaging metrics performed in Chapter 2, dFNC analysis of fMRI data was done to compare the differences between CBS and PSP patient groups under two resting state (RS) conditions of eyes closing (RS EC) and physiological unconscious (RS PH) situations. Same connectogram nodes were chosen including the six important functional networks, and results of two representative states such as connectogram and correlation matrix as well as occurrence, frequency and dwell time parameters of all states (six for our data) were illustrated for dynamic comparison between two patient sub-groups as well as between RS EC and RS PH conditions.

2.2. CBF with ASL and ADSP PHC Composite Score

MRI imaging and clinical data used in the preparation of this section were obtained from the Alzheimer's Disease Neuroimaging Initiative (ADNI) database (http://ida.loni.usc.edu) with approval. The primary goal of ADNI has been to test whether serial MRI, positron emission tomography (PET), other biological markers, and clinical and neuropsychological assessment can be combined to measure the progression of mild cognitive impairment (MCI) and early Alzheimer's disease (AD). ADNI is the result of efforts of many co-investigators from a broad range of academic institutions and private corporations, and subjects have been recruited from over 50 sites across the United States and Canada. For up-to- date information, see www.adni-info.org.

The relatively new cerebral blood flow (CBF) data acquired with arterial spin labeling (ASL) sequence was processed at the Center for Imaging of Neurodegenerative Diseases (CIND) as one of the ADNI featured center. Region of interest (ROI)-based CBF computation utilized several software packages such as SPM8 (Statistical Parametric Mapping, http://www.fil.ion.ucl.ac.uk), EPI nonlinear geometric distortion correction via FSL commands (FMRIB Software Library, http://www.fmrib.ox.ac.uk/fsl), FreeSurfer (http://surfer.nmr.mgh.harvard.edu), Insight Toolkit (ITK, http://itk.org) and MATLAB (www.mathworks.com) scripts. The

CBF processing pipeline included: 1) motion correction of the individual ASL frames (realignment in SPM); 2) computation of the perfusion-weighted imaging (PWI) by subtracting the mean of tagged from untagged ASL data sets; 3) alignment of ASL and structural MRI data (co-registration); 4) geometric distortion correction; 5) partial volume correction; and 6) CBF quantification in physical units by normalizing ASL to an estimated blood water density signal with ROI segmented from standardized anatomical MRI data [43-47].

Neuropsychological batteries might differ across various cohorts, and standard composite scores in different studies that might be assessed with several test batteries were needed for post-hoc data analysis and integration. The co-calibration or centralization of memory (MEM), executive function (EXF), language (LAN), and visuospatial processing (VSP) composite scores across four cohorts were performed including ADNI, Adult Changes in Thought (ACT), the Religious Orders Study and the Memory and Aging Project (ROS/MAP), and the National Alzheimer's Coordinating Center (NACC). The AD Sequencing Project (ADSP)-phenotype harmonization consortium (PHC) co-calibrated scores of each metric were further standardized so that these composite scores could be directly comparable across center to account for any possible test-administration differences, and were usable to correlate with imaging results [48-49].

A total of 20 early AD (age: 76.7 ± 1.7 years), 43 MCI (age: 74.7 ± 1.3 years) and 78 controls (age: 73.6 ± 0.9 years) were selected for between-group comparison of CBF data as well as correlation with ADSP-PHC composite scores.

2.3. PET and MRI Correlation in Asymptotic AD

The Anti-Amyloid Treatment in Asymptomatic Alzheimer's study (the A4 Study for short) is a landmark of public-private partnership, funded by the National Institute on Aging/NIH, Eli Lilly and Company, and several philanthropic organizations. The A4 trial is coordinated by the University of Southern California's Alzheimer's Therapeutic Research Institute, with study sites in multiple locations and is one primary ADNI center. MRI and PET data from 327 Aβ+ and 935 Aβ- asymptomatic participants were selected, compared and correlated for each ROI from the A4 data cohort.

The PET amyloid imaging with standardized uptake value ratio (SUVR) values greater than or equal to 1.15 was considered Aβ+ for enrolled participants (cut-off value = 1.15, with cerebellar reference) [50, 51]. Seven ROIs were quantified for PET SUVR amyloid accumulation: xlaal_frontal_med_orb = frontal cortex, new_temporal_2 = temporal cortex, lprecuneus_gm = precuneus, lnew_parietal = parietal cortex, llposterior_cingulate_2 = posterior cingulate, lanterior_cingulate_2 = anterior cingulate, Composite_Summary = composite summary.

The 3D T1-weighted MRI images were processed and quantitative regional volumetry was obtained using the NeuroQuant (NQ) package (http://www.cortechslabs.com/neuroquant), an automated segmentation software approved for clinical use. Quality control to check for severe patient motion and other artifacts, personalized age- and gender- specific atlas for each subject, together with automated segmentation and volume calculation in individual space were three primary steps involved in NQ software [52]. Finally, the hippocampal occupancy (HOC) score was computed as the ratio of hippocampal volume to the sum of hippocampal and inferior lateral ventricle volumes to generate the medial temporal atrophy index.

3. RESULTS

3.1. DFNC Application in CBS and PSP under RS EC Condition

Under the RS EC condition, representative networks in CBS and PSP patients including DMN and VN were demonstrated in Figure 2. Decreased VN connectivity but increased frontal DMN were observed in PSP patients compared to CBS group with ICA decomposition. A total of six typical networks including DMN, FPN, SN, MN, VN and CEN (EN) were used for the dFNC analysis with GIFT software. Figure 3 illustrated the connectogram of two representative states of S3 and S4 in both CBS (Figure 3; panel A1 and A2) and PSP patients (panel B1 and B2). Hypo-connectivity between SN and CEN, between FPN and CEN, DMN and VN were identified comparing PSP to CBS at S3 state (Figure 3; panel B1 and A1). In contrast, hyper-connectivity between FPN and DMN, between MN and VN were present in PSP compared to CBS at S3 condition as well.

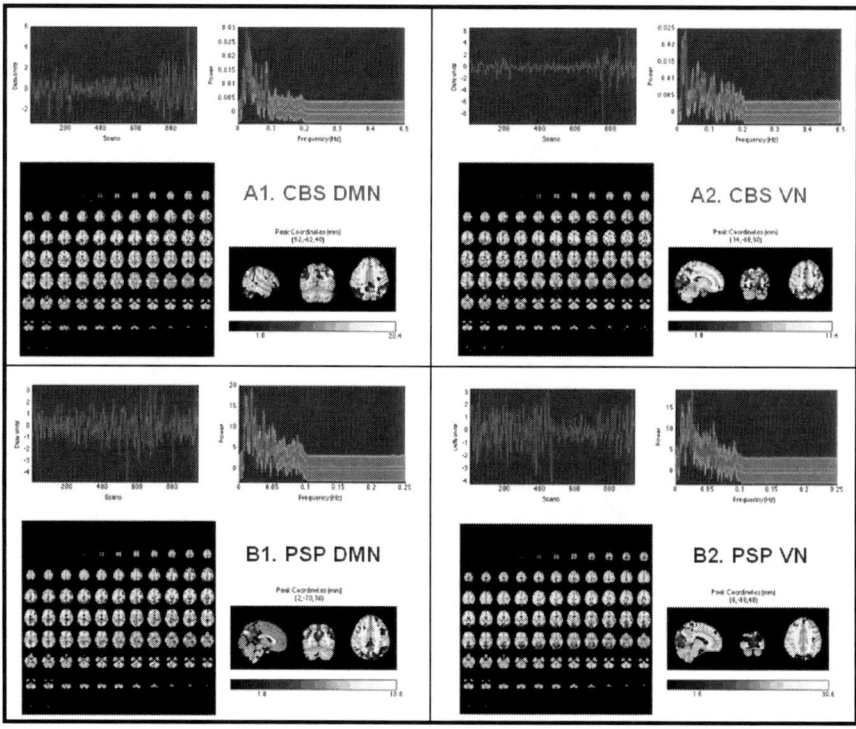

Figure 2. Representative networks in CBS and PSP patients including DMN and VN at the conventional resting state closing eyes (RS EC) condition. A1: Upper panel showed the averaged time course and power spectrum of this specific ICA component, with periodic temporal wave and power spectrum centered in the low frequency of around 0.03 Hz. Lower panel showed the spatial distribution of the ICA component in multi-slice and 3-orientation views. Based on the spatial distribution and distinct power peak, this component was most likely to be default mode network (DMN). Similarly, visual network (VN) was identified based on the spatial pattern and low-frequency fluctuation in A2. Decreased visual network connectivity but increased frontal DMN were observed in PSP patients compared to CBS group with ICA decomposition as shown in B1 and B2.

At state S4, hypo-connectivity between MN and VN, FPN and DMN, SN and MN were found comparing PSP to CBS; but hyper-connectivity between VN and CEN, MN and CEN, DMN and SN existed in PSP as well. Overall, PSP group had less inter-network correlation such as less SN and CEN dFNC compared to CBS patients.

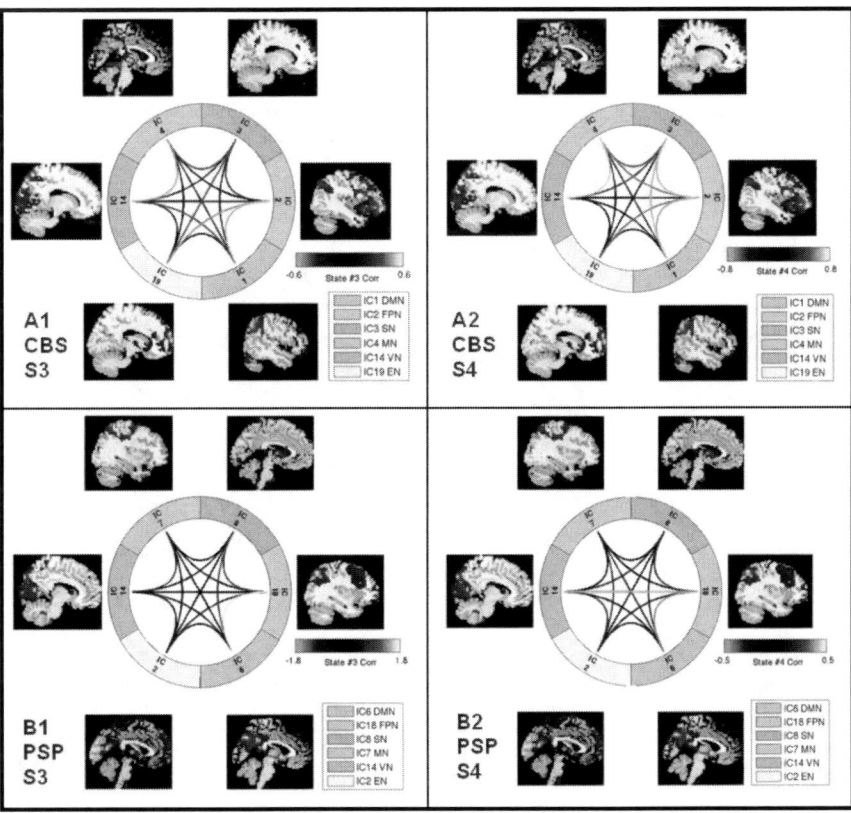

Figure 3. Connectogram of representative states S3 and S4 in CBS (panel A1 and A2) and PSP patients (panel B1 and B2). Dynamic hypo-connectivity between SN and CEN, between FPN and CEN, DMN and VN were identified comparing PSP to CBS at S3 state under RS EC condition (panel B1 and A1). In contrast, hyper-connectivity between FPN and DMN, between MN and VN were present in PSP compared to CBS at S3 condition. At state S4, hypo-connectivity between MN and VN, FPN and DMN, SN and MN were found comparing PSP to CBS; but hyper-connectivity between VN and CEN, MN and CEN, DMN and SN existed in PSP as well. Overall, less inter-network correlation in PSP compared to CBS patients was illustrated in the connectogram. Largely, lower SN and CEN dFNC in PSP compared to CBS participants were identified.

Furthermore, the inter-network dFNC correlation matrix (from six networks) of states S3 and S4 in CBS (panel A1 and A2) and PSP patients (panel B1 and B2) were derived respectively (Figure 4), with a sliding-window size of default value (22 TRs=44 sec). The percentage of occurrence in state S3 was lower in PSP compared to CBS (3% in PSP vs. 11% in CBS), but increased slightly at state 4 in PSP (22% in PSP vs. 18% in CBS).

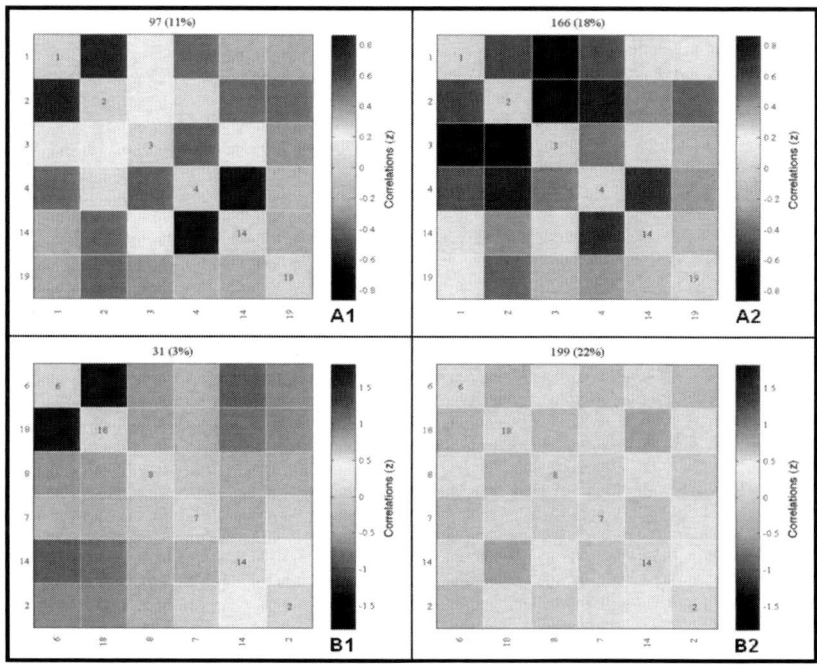

Figure 4. dFNC correlation matrix of state S3 and S4 in CBS (panel A1 and A2) and PSP patients (panel B1 and B2) respectively. The percentage of occurrence in S3 was lower in PSP compared to CBS (3% in PSP vs. 11% in CBS), but increased slightly at state S4 in PSP (22% in PSP vs. 18% in CBS).

Figure 5 also displayed the cluster occurrence distribution along the dynamic time range for six states (S1-S6) in CBS (A) and PSP (B) groups. In addition to previous changes in states S3 and S4 of PSP compared to CBS, the percentage of occurrence in S1 was increased in PSP compared to CBS (15% vs. 9%) but slightly changes in S5 and S6 states in two groups (4-5% differences), with less state dynamics revealed in PSP.

Novel Imaging Biomarkers in CBS/PSP ...

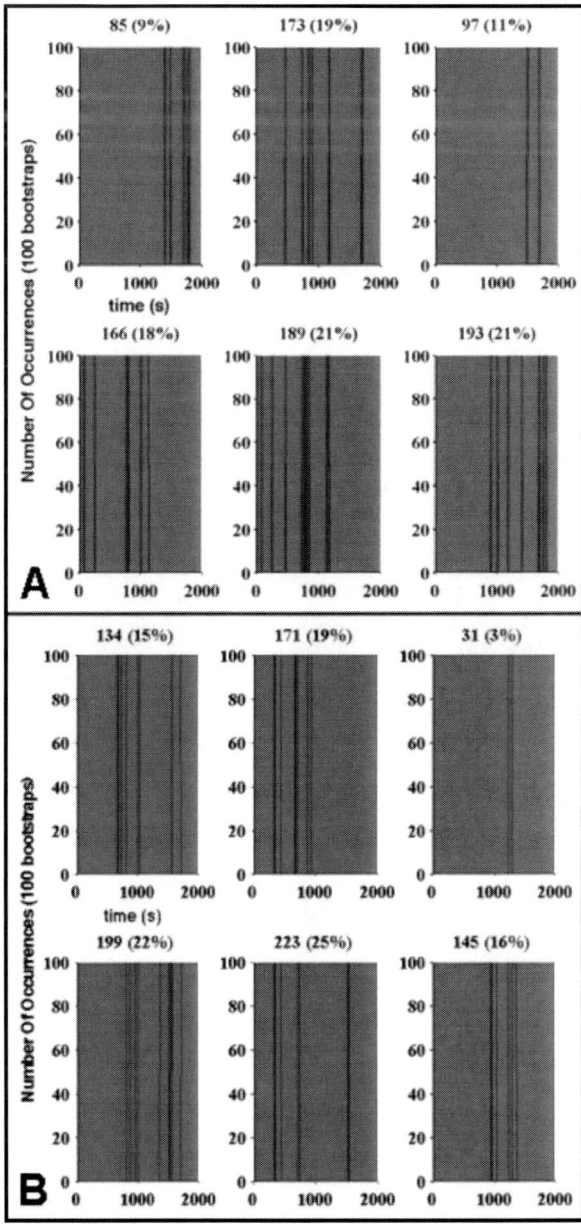

Figure 5. Cluster occurrence distribution along the dynamic time range in six states (S1-S6) in CBS (A) and PSP (B) groups. In addition to previous changes in states S3 and S4, the percentage of occurrence in S1 was increased in PSP compared to CBS (15% vs. 9%), and slightly changes in S5 and S6 states in PSP compared to CBS (4-5% differences) together with less overall dynamics revealed.

Also based on the frequency and mean dell time of sliding windows for all states, PSP patients had lower frequency in states 3 and 6 but higher frequency in states 1, 4 and 5 than CBS group (Figure 6). In addition, PSP patients spent much less time (lower dwell time in units of window) in states 3 and 4 but more time in states 1 and 5 compared to CBS group.

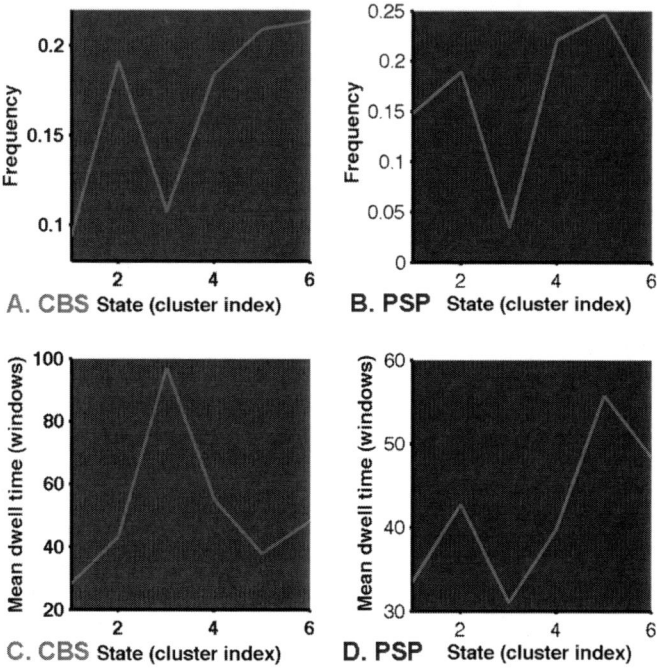

Figure 6. Frequency and mean dell time in CBS (left panel - A and C respectively) as well as in PSP patients (right panel - B and D). PSP Patients had less frequency in states 3 and 6 but more frequency in states 1, 4 and 5 than CBS. PSP also spent much less time in states 3 and 4 but more time in states 1 and 5 with overall lower dell time.

3.2. DFNC Application in CBS and PSP under RS PH Condition

Under the RS PH condition, both DMN and VN connectives were decreased in CBS patients compared to RS EC condition (Figure 7). However, in PSP patients, DMN and VN increased slightly including the pericalcarine region and medial prefrontal cortex. Overall, under RS PH condition, intra- DMN and VN connectivities were higher in PSP compared to CBS patients. Connectogram of representative states S3 and S4 in CBS and PSP patients under RS PH condition were demonstrated in Figure 8. Hypo-connectivity between SN and FPN, SN and CEN but hyper-connectivity between VN and CEN, VN and FPN, VN and DMN were present in PSP compared to CBS at state S3. On the other hand, hypo-connectivity between DMN and SN, DMN and MN, DMN and VN but hyper-connectivity between DMN and CEN were identified at state S4. Overall, lower SN dFNC was observed in PSP compared to CBS.

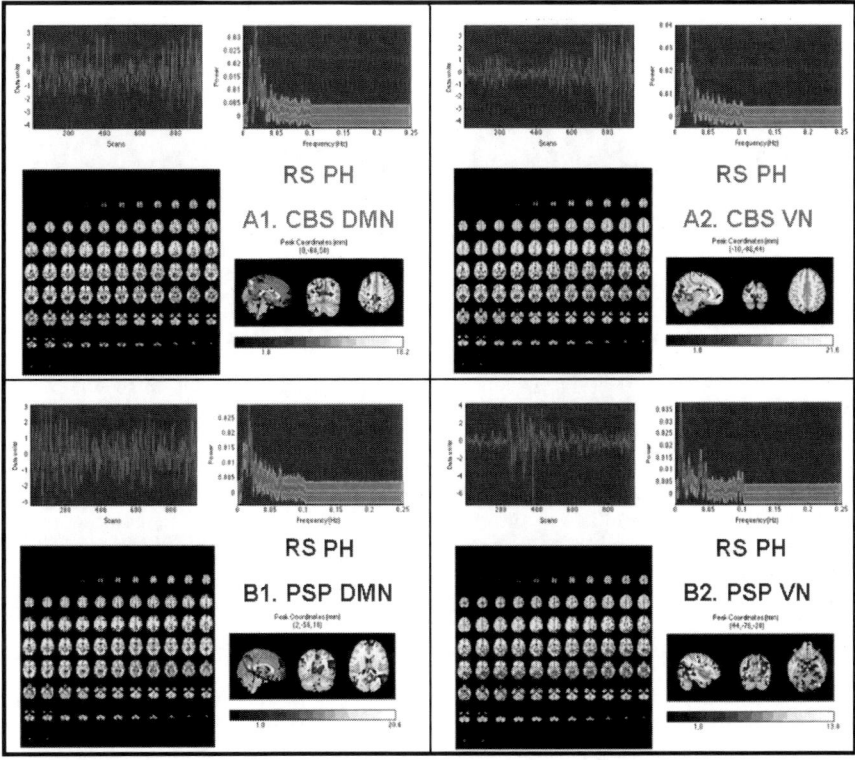

Figure 7. Under the RS PH condition, both DMN and VN dynamic connectives were decreased in CBS patients compared to RS EC condition as expected. However in PSP patients, DMN and VN increased slightly including the pericalcarine region and medial prefrontal cortex. Overall, DMN and VN connectivities were higher in PSP compared to CBS patients under RS PH condition.

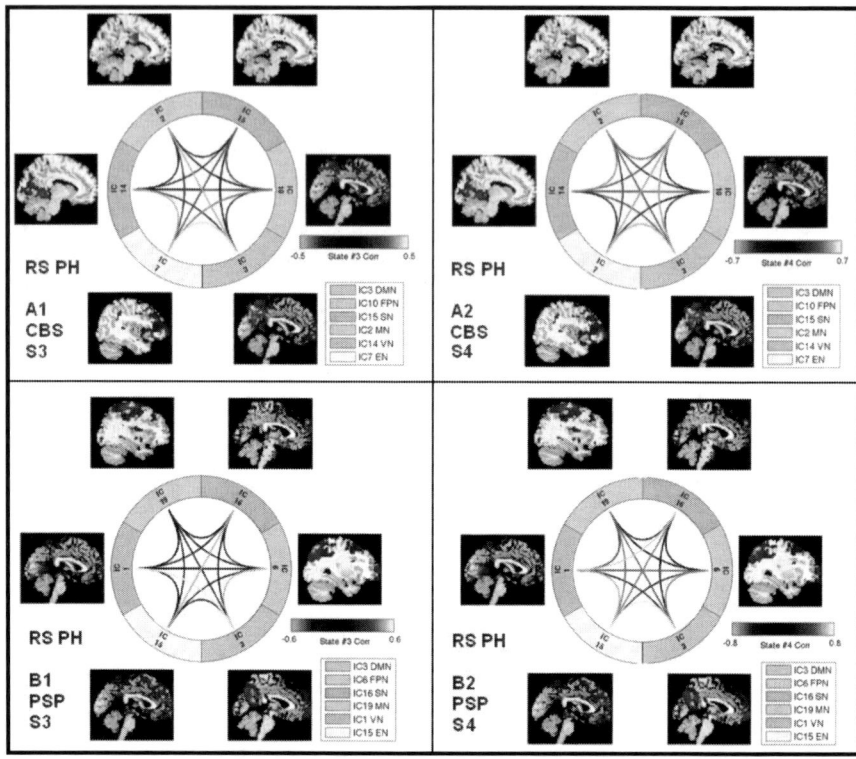

Figure 8. Connectogram of representative states S3 and S4 in CBS (panel A1 and A2) and PSP patients (panel B1 and B2) under RS PH condition. Hypo-connectivity between FPN and SN, SN and CEN but hyper-connectivity between VN and CEN, FPN and VN, DMN and VN were present in PSP compared to CBS at S3 state. At state S4, hypo-connectivity between DMN and SN, DMN and MN, DMN and VN but hyper-connectivity between DMN and CEN were identified on the other hand. Lower SN dFNC in PSP compared to CBS existed generally.

Based on the dFNC correlation matrices, the percentages of occurrence in two states were quite close in both patient groups (~18%) with different correlation strengths among six networks (Figure 9). For the other states as illustrated in Figure 10, the percentage of occurrence in S6 was increased in PSP compared to CBS (30% vs. 13%), but decreased in S2 (6% vs. 16%) and S5 (17% vs. 24%) in PSP compared to CBS. Also PSP patients had lower frequency in states 2 and 5 but higher frequency in states 4 and 6 than CBS. In contrast to the RS EC condition, PSP patients spent more time in majority of states including S1, S3, S5 and 6, with less time in states 2 and 4 than CBS (Figure 11). In summary, similar to the RS EC condition, the PSP patients presented less dynamics with smaller number of dynamic transitions than CBS patients under the RS PH condition.

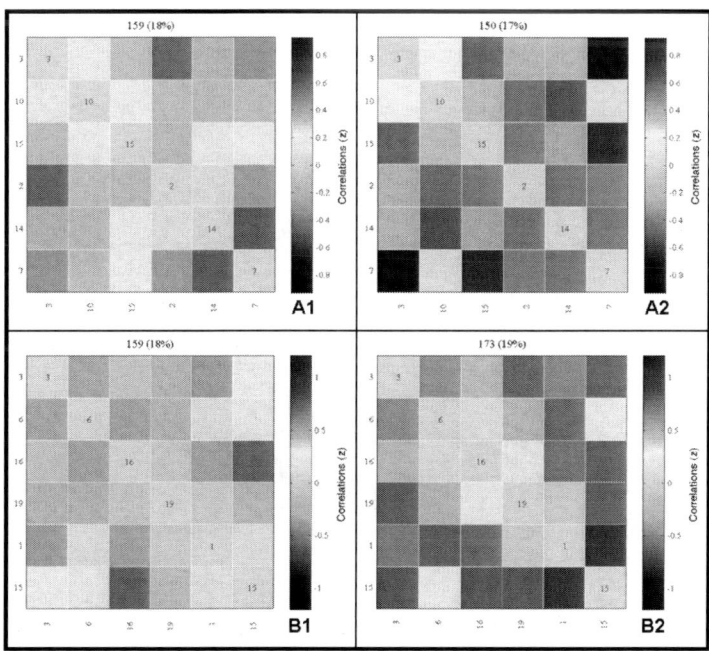

Figure 9. dFNC correlation matrix of states S3 and S4 in CBS (panel A1 and A2) and PSP patients (panel B1 and B2) respectively. The percentages of occurrence in two states were quite close in both patient groups (~18%).

3.3. CBF Comparisons and Correlation in MCI/AD

In nine ROIs that presented significantly lower CBF based on MRI ASL sequence in MCI and AD patients compared to controls (except for ROI-cbf34, P = 0.09 comparing MCI to NC), lowest CBF values were observed in AD patients with P < 0.01 (Figure 12). However, no significant differences between MCI and AD groups were found for these listed ROIs (except P = 0.02 comparing AD to MCI for ROI-cbf59). Using the composite cognitive scores from the ADSP-PHC, significantly lower scores in the four domains of memory, executive function, language and visuospatial processing were found in AD patients compared to both controls (NC) and MCI (P < 0.001 for most tests; except P = 0.16

comparing PHC_VSP score of MCI to AD) (Figure 13). Relatively lower scores in MCI compared to NC group were found in three tests as well (P < 0.001 except P = 0.03 for PHC_VSP test).

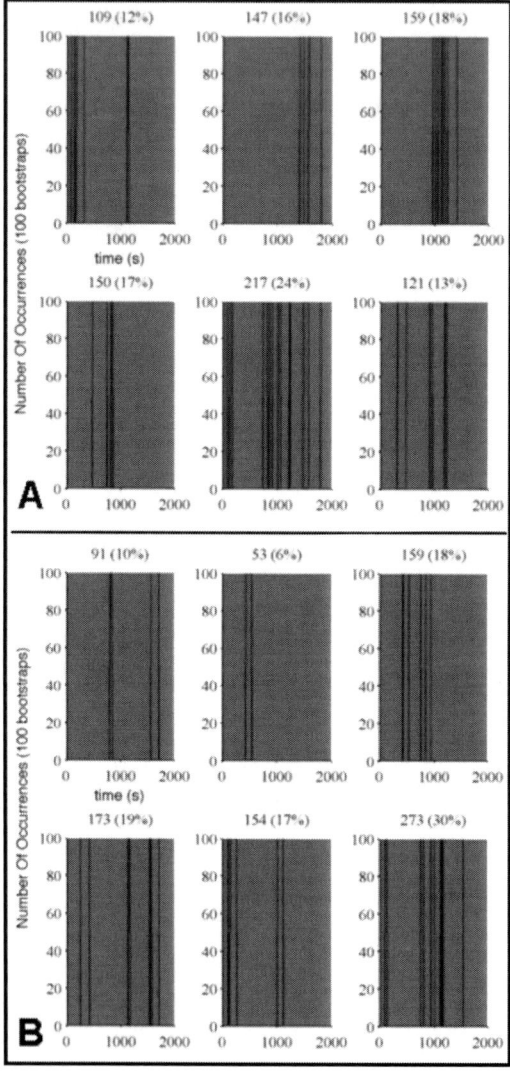

Figure 10. Cluster occurrence distribution along the dynamic time range in six states (S1-S6) in CBS (A) and PSP (B) groups under RS PH condition of states S1 and S5 in CBS (panel A) and PSP patients (panel B) respectively. The percentage of occurrence in S6 was increased in PSP compared to CBS (30% vs. 13%), but decreased in S2 (6% vs. 16%) and S5 in PSP compared to CBS (17% vs. 24%) with less overall dynamics.

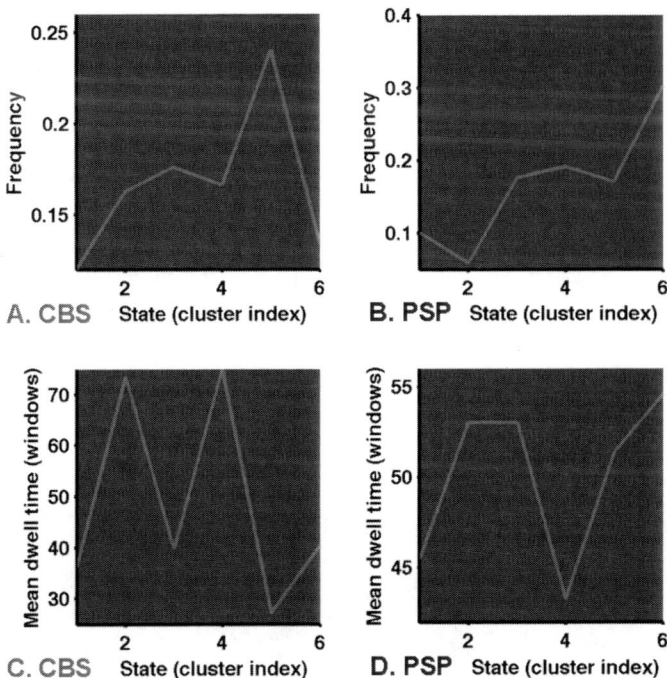

Figure 11. Frequency and mean dell time in CBS (left panel - A and C respectively) as well as in PSP patients (right panel - B and D) under RS PH condition. PSP Patients had less frequency in states 2 and 5 but more frequency in states 4 and 6 than CBS. PSP patients spent less time in states 2 and 4 but more time in states 1, 3, 5 and 6 than CBS.

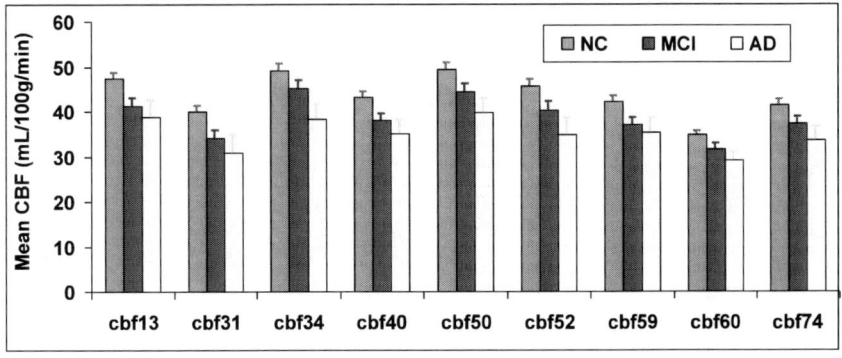

Figure 12. Significantly lower CBF in MCI and AD patients compared to controls ($P < 0.05$) for most ROIs listed (except $P = 0.09$ for ROI-cbf34 between MCI and NC). Lowest CBF values were observed in AD patients with $P < 0.01$ between AD and NC for most listed ROIs (except $P = 0.02$ for ROI-cbf59); however, no significant differences between MCI and AD groups.

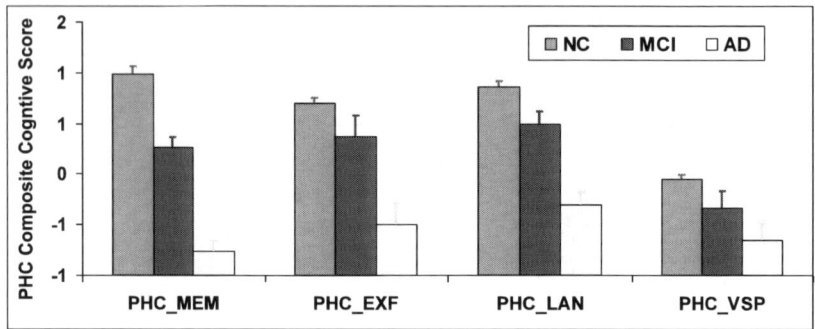

Figure 13. Significantly lower composite cognitive score from the ADSP phenotype harmonization consortium (PHC) in AD compared to NC and MCI (P < 0.001 for most tests except P = 0.16 for PHC_VSP comparing MCI to AD), as well as lower score in MCI compared to NC (P < 0.001 except P = 0.03 for PHC_VSP test).

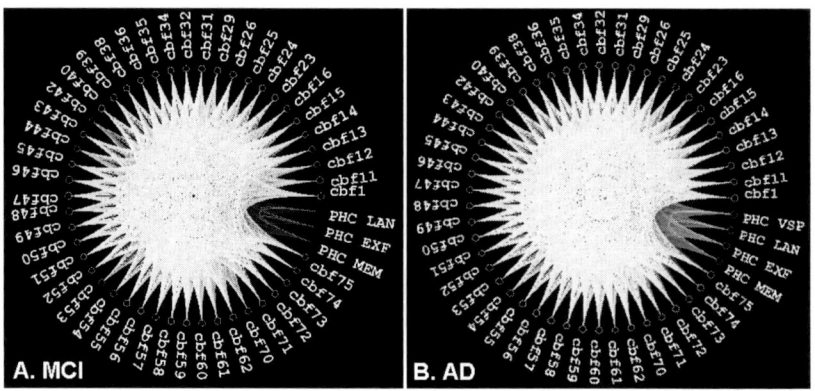

Figure 14. Significant intra- and inter- correlations of CBF and composite cognitive scores in MCI and AD patients (P < 0.01, r>0.35). Mild negative correlations between CBF and cognitive scores in MCI but positive correlations in AD were observed in A and B respectively.

Significant correlations between regional CBF measured and quantified with MRI ASL sequence and composite scores in domains of memory and language function ($|r|>0.23$, $P < 0.05$) are listed in Table 1. The representative significant intra- and inter- correlations between CBF and composite cognitive scores in MCI and AD patients (P < 0.01, r>0.35) were demonstrated in Figure 14 circle plot. Mild negative correlations between CBF and cognitive composite scores in MCI but positive correlations in AD were observed in Figure 14A and B respectively.

Table 1. Significant correlations between ROI-based CBF measured and quantified with MRI ASL sequence and ADSP phenotype harmonization consortium (PHC) cognitive tests such as memory (PHC_MEM) and language function (PHC_LAN) ($|r|>0.23$, $P < 0.05$)

ROI	Cognitive tests	r	p
Control Group			
cbf14	PHC_MEM	0.2326	0.0405
cbf23	PHC_MEM	0.2353	0.0381
cbf25	PHC_MEM	0.2346	0.0387
cbf26	PHC_MEM	0.2688	0.0173
cbf31	PHC_MEM	0.2300	0.0428
cbf32	PHC_MEM	0.2310	0.0418
cbf34	PHC_MEM	0.2672	0.0180
cbf35	PHC_MEM	0.2403	0.0341
cbf38	PHC_MEM	0.2629	0.0201
cbf43	PHC_MEM	0.2481	0.0285
cbf44	PHC_MEM	0.2835	0.0119
cbf48	PHC_MEM	0.2434	0.0317
cbf50	PHC_MEM	0.3235	0.0039
cbf52	PHC_MEM	0.2747	0.0149
cbf57	PHC_MEM	0.2490	0.0279
MCI Group			
cbf11	PHC_MEM	-0.3733	0.0137
cbf42	PHC_MEM	-0.4248	0.0045
cbf53	PHC_MEM	-0.4315	0.0039
cbf70	PHC_MEM	-0.3762	0.0129
cbf75	PHC_MEM	-0.3393	0.0260
AD Group			
cbf11	PHC_MEM	0.4930	0.0272
cbf50	PHC_MEM	0.4456	0.0490
cbf11	PHC_LAN	0.5092	0.0219
cbf12	PHC_LAN	0.4553	0.0437
cbf70	PHC_LAN	0.5063	0.0227
cbf71	PHC_LAN	0.4464	0.0485

3.4. MRI and PET Differences and Correlations of Aβ+ vs. Aβ- Groups

Significantly higher amyloid deposition in all seven brain regions comparing asymptomatic Aβ+ to Aβ- carriers ($P < 0.00001$) was confirmed as shown in Figure 15, including both anterior and posterior cingulate, precuneus, parietal, temporal and media-orbito frontal lobes and global composite brain area. Moreover, in Aβ+ carriers, negative associations between regional volume measured with MRI volumetry and amyloid accumulation using PET amyloid tracer were observed. Particularly, significant correlations between temporal/parietal MRI volume and cingulate/media-orbito frontal amyloid deposition in these asymptomatic sample ($|r|>0.14$, $P < 0.01$) are listed in Table 2. Representative strong intra- and inter- correlations ($P < 0.001$) between MRI volumetry and PET amyloid SUVR are also illustrated in the circle plot in Figure 16.

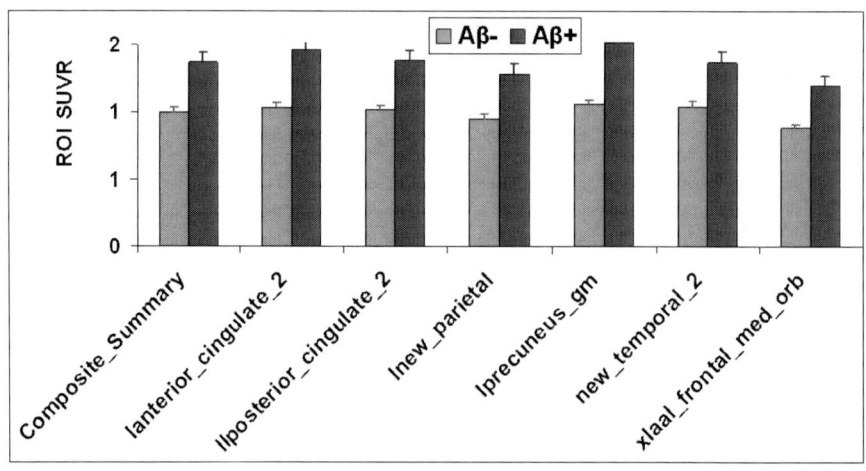

Figure 15. Illustration of significantly higher amyloid deposition in all seven brain regions comparing asymptomatic Aβ+ to Aβ- carriers ($P < 0.00001$). xlaal_frontal_med_orb = frontal cortex, new_temporal_2 = temporal cortex, lprecuneus_gm = precuneus, lnew_parietal = parietal cortex, llposterior_cingulate_2 = posterior cingulate, lanterior_cingulate_2 = anterior cingulate.

Table 2. Most significant correlations between regional volume and amyloid accumulation in asymptomatic Aβ+ carriers measured with MRI volumetry and PET amyloid tracer (|r|>0.14, P < 0.01)

MRI Volume	PET Amyloid SUVR	r	P
Left Hippocampus	lanterior_cingulate_2	-0.1514	0.0061
Left Amygdala	lanterior_cingulate_2	-0.1564	0.0046
Right Ventral Diencephalon	lanterior_cingulate_2	-0.1451	0.0086
Right Inferior Parietal	lanterior_cingulate_2	-0.1478	0.0074
Left Temporal Pole	lanterior_cingulate_2	-0.1537	0.0054
Right Inferior Parietal	llposterior_cingulate_2	-0.1426	0.0098
Right Inferior Parietal	xlaal_frontal_med_orb	-0.1594	0.0038
Left Temporal Pole	xlaal_frontal_med_orb	-0.1614	0.0034

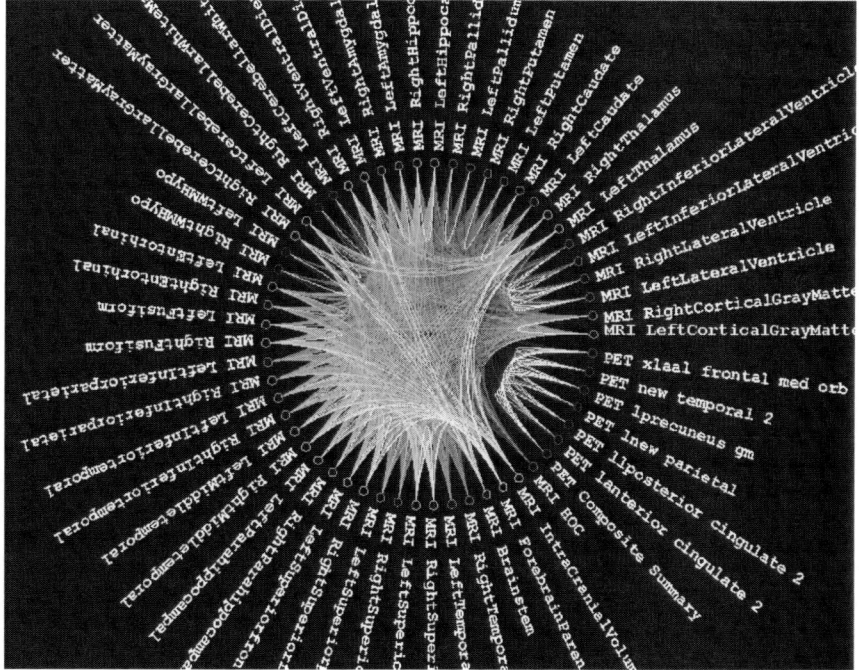

Figure 16. Representative strong intra- and inter- correlations of MRI volumetry and PET amyloid SUVR (P ≪ 0.01) in Aβ+ carriers.

4. DISCUSSION

4.1. Summary of Results

In this work, we had reported the dynamic FNC differences between CBS and PSP patients under both RS EC and RS PH conditions, and revealed the lower temporal dynamics in PSP compared to CBS. Specifically, state-dependent connectivity changes in two groups such as lower SN and MN, but higher VN dFNC in PSP compared to CBS under RS PH condition together with lower CEN and SN dFNC in PSP under RS EC condition were illustrated. The results of different connectivity patterns under two conditions were similar to previous findings of VMHC and ICA-DR as well as DTI results reported in Chapter 2. For instance, under RS EC condition, lower SN and CEN dynamic transitions with dFNC method were in agreement with the hypo-network modulation using ICA-DR algorithm in PSP compared to CBS participants. Also under RS PH condition, lower SN dFNC in PSP compared to CBS was similar to the ICA-DR inter-network modulation and RS EC dFNC finding. Disruption of SN dynamics under both RS conditions was probably related to the disinhibition function that was common to both PD subtypes, and state/attention shifting role of SN. Observations of abnormal interhemispheric conductivity, white matter micro-structural connectivity deterioration, inter-network dis-coordination and less temporal dynamics under two RS conditions were consistent, and indicated possible spatiotemporal communication and state-dependent pathway distortion at different degrees in two patient cohorts.

Moreover, we found significantly lower ASL-CBF values in MCI/AD patients compared to controls ($P < 0.05$) for most ROIs, and slightly lower in AD compared to MCI. Strong correlations in multiple brain regions between CBF and memory composite score were present more in controls, less in MCI and AD patients. Moreover, only in AD, CBF in a few regions correlated with language composite score. Also significant correlations between amyloid deposition in the anterior cingulate/medial orbitofrontal ROI and MRI temporoparietal volume were identified in asymptomatic

Aβ+ carriers. The combination of these novel imaging metrics such as dFNC and ASL-CBF together with conventional imaging quantifications could improve disease detection and help interpret transit changes between brain states at regular physiological conditions in patients.

4.2. Relating to Other Published Works

The temporal features of fMRI signal, especially characterizing the changes in macroscopic neural activity patterns using dFNC metrics, contained rich information about brain cognition and behavior [53]. There existed dFNC differences between resting and task conditions; for instance, positive CEN-SN connectivity occurred more frequently during task than rest [54]. Based on a recent study, the cross domain mutual information (CDMI) was strong in the subcortical domain, while the high-level cortical cognitive regions had a different pattern with much less information sharing across domains [55]. On a developmental view, sensorimotor areas were reported to be the most active, well-connected and temporally dynamic region in neonates; while visual and primary auditory areas had higher or similar local activity but with lower static and dynamic connections [56].

Time-varying dynamic fALFF (neural activity marker) was found to be associated with dFNC, with both showing alterations in disease and might disrupt brain cognitive function [57]. Also dFNC methods could be used to predict treatment outcome; for instance, dFNC between DMN and antinociceptive system mediated the variability of links between temporal summation of pain and treatment effects [58]. In stroke patients, severity of patients was related to the dwell time of a densely connected and isolated brain state, and dFNC involving DMN configuration correlated with recovery poststroke [59]. The psychopathy traits were associated with FNC and dFNC quantifications, including positive correlation between impulsive/antisocial behaviors scores and dynamic variables [60]. dFNC was also found to be connected with genetics and clinical measures in Huntington's disease, with less dynamism in patients compared to healthy controls [61]. In major depressive disorder, several dFNCs involving lower centrality nodes such as parietal lobule, lingual gyrus and thalamus had aberrant patterns, and were correlated with depressive symptom severity and cognitive performance [62].

In conclusion, the dFNC results presented in this chapter complemented typical imaging findings of CBS and PSP patients as in previous chapter, with consistent dynamic connectogram results such as less overall transitions in PSP compared to CBS. Distinguishable dFNC patterns at RS PH and RS EC situations were also in agreement with the multiparametric VMHC/ICA-DR/DTI results of Chapter 2. Furthermore, these imaging metrics including interhemispheric conductivity deficit, white matter micro-structural connectivity deterioration, inter-network discoordination and less temporal dynamics in PSP compared to CBS implicated both static and dynamic systematic deficits at multiple scales for two atypical Parkinsonism.

REFERENCES

[1] Calhoun VD, Miller R, Pearlson G, Adalı T. The chronnectome: time-varying connectivity networks as the next frontier in fMRI data discovery. *Neuron.* 2014 Oct 22;84(2):262-74. doi: 10.1016/j.neuron.2014.10.015. Epub 2014 Oct 22. PMID: 25374354; PMCID: PMC4372723.

[2] Allen EA, Damaraju E, Plis SM, Erhardt EB, Eichele T, Calhoun VD. Tracking whole-brain connectivity dynamics in the resting state. *Cereb Cortex.* 2014 Mar;24(3):663-76. doi: 10.1093/cercor/bhs352. Epub 2012 Nov 11. PMID: 23146964; PMCID: PMC3920766.

[3] Miller RL, Yaesoubi M, Calhoun VD. Higher dimensional analysis shows reduced dynamism of time-varying network connectivity in schizophrenia patients. *Annu Int Conf IEEE Eng Med Biol Soc.* 2014;2014:3837-40. doi: 10.1109/EMBC.2014.6944460. PMID: 25570828.

[4] Faghiri A, Damaraju E, Belger A, Ford JM, Mathalon D, McEwen S, Mueller B, Pearlson G, Preda A, Turner JA, Vaidya JG, Van Erp T, Calhoun VD. Brain Density Clustering Analysis: A New Approach to Brain Functional Dynamics. *Front Neurosci.* 2021 Apr 13;15:621716. doi: 10.3389/fnins.2021.621716. PMID: 33927587; PMCID: PMC8076753.

[5] Liégeois R, Laumann TO, Snyder AZ, Zhou J, Yeo BTT. Interpreting temporal fluctuations in resting-state functional connectivity MRI. *Neuroimage.* 2017 Dec;163:437-455. doi: 10.1016/j.neuroimage.2017.09.012. Epub 2017 Sep 12. PMID: 28916180.

[6] Zhou Y. *Joint Imaging Applications in General Neurodegenerative Disease: Parkinson's, Frontotemporal, Vascular Dementia and Autism.* Nova Science Publishers. 2021.

[7] Zhou Y. *Functional Neuroimaging Methods and Frontiers.* Nova Science Publishers. 2018.

[8] Preti MG, Bolton TA, Van De Ville D. The dynamic functional connectome: State-of-the-art and perspectives. *Neuroimage.* 2017 Oct 15;160:41-54. doi: 10.1016/j.neuroimage.2016.12.061. Epub 2016 Dec 26. PMID: 28034766.

[9] Fu Z, Du Y, Calhoun VD. The Dynamic Functional Network Connectivity Analysis Framework. *Engineering* (Beijing). 2019 Apr;5(2):190-193. doi: 10.1016/j.eng.2018.10.001. Epub 2018 Oct 24. PMID: 32489683; PMCID: PMC7265753.

[10] Hindriks R, Adhikari MH, Murayama Y, Ganzetti M, Mantini D, Logothetis NK, Deco G. Can sliding-window correlations reveal dynamic functional connectivity in resting-state fMRI? *Neuroimage.* 2016 Feb 15;127:242-256. doi: 10.1016/j.neuroimage.2015.11.055. Epub 2015 Nov 26. Erratum in: Neuroimage. 2016 May 15;132:115. PMID: 26631813; PMCID: PMC4758830.

[11] Lurie DJ, Kessler D, Bassett DS, Betzel RF, Breakspear M, Kheilholz S, Kucyi A, Liégeois R, Lindquist MA, McIntosh AR, Poldrack RA, Shine JM, Thompson WH, Bielczyk NZ, Douw L, Kraft D, Miller RL, Muthuraman M, Pasquini L, Razi A, Vidaurre D, Xie H, Calhoun VD. Questions and controversies in the study of

time-varying functional connectivity in resting fMRI. *Netw Neurosci.* 2020 Feb 1;4(1):30-69. doi: 10.1162/netn_a_00116. PMID: 32043043; PMCID: PMC7006871.

[12] Choe AS, Nebel MB, Barber AD, Cohen JR, Xu Y, Pekar JJ, Caffo B, Lindquist MA. Comparing test-retest reliability of dynamic functional connectivity methods. *Neuroimage.* 2017 Sep;158:155-175. doi: 10.1016/j.neuroimage.2017.07.005. Epub 2017 Jul 5. PMID: 28687517; PMCID: PMC5614828.

[13] Baker BT, Damaraju E, Silva RF, Plis SM, Calhoun VD. Decentralized dynamic functional network connectivity: State analysis in collaborative settings. *Hum Brain Mapp.* 2020 Aug 1;41(11):2909-2925. doi: 10.1002/hbm.24986. Epub 2020 Apr 21. PMID: 32319193; PMCID: PMC7336163.

[14] Liang L, Yuan Y, Wei Y, Yu B, Mai W, Duan G, Nong X, Li C, Su J, Zhao L, Zhang Z, Deng D. Recurrent and concurrent patterns of regional BOLD dynamics and functional connectivity dynamics in cognitive decline. *Alzheimers Res Ther.* 2021 Jan 16;13(1):28. doi: 10.1186/s13195-020-00764-6. PMID: 33453729; PMCID: PMC7811744.

[15] Allen EA, Damaraju E, Eichele T, Wu L, Calhoun VD. EEG Signatures of Dynamic Functional Network Connectivity States. *Brain Topogr.* 2018 Jan;31(1):101-116. doi: 10.1007/s10548-017-0546-2. Epub 2017 Feb 22. PMID: 28229308; PMCID: PMC 5568463.

[16] Zhou S, Zou G, Xu J, Su Z, Zhu H, Zou Q, Gao JH. Dynamic functional connectivity states characterize NREM sleep and wakefulness. *Hum Brain Mapp.* 2019 Dec 15;40(18):5256-5268. doi: 10.1002/hbm.24770. Epub 2019 Aug 24. PMID: 31444893; PMCID: PMC6865216.

[17] Wilson RS, Mayhew SD, Rollings DT, Goldstone A, Przezdzik I, Arvanitis TN, Bagshaw AP. Influence of epoch length on measurement of dynamic functional connectivity in wakefulness and behavioural validation in sleep. *Neuroimage.* 2015 May 15;112:169-

179. doi: 10.1016/j.neuroimage.2015.02.061. Epub 2015 Mar 10. PMID: 25765256.

[18] Du Y, Fu Z, Calhoun VD. Classification and Prediction of Brain Disorders Using Functional Connectivity: Promising but Challenging. *Front Neurosci.* 2018 Aug 6;12:525. doi: 10.3389/fnins.2018.00525. PMID: 30127711; PMCID: PMC6088208.

[19] Du Y, Pearlson GD, Lin D, Sui J, Chen J, Salman M, Tamminga CA, Ivleva EI, Sweeney JA, Keshavan MS, Clementz BA, Bustillo J, Calhoun VD. Identifying dynamic functional connectivity biomarkers using GIG-ICA: Application to schizophrenia, schizoaffective disorder, and psychotic bipolar disorder. *Hum Brain Mapp.* 2017 May;38(5):2683-2708. doi: 10.1002/hbm.23553. Epub 2017 Mar 10. PMID: 28294459; PMCID: PMC5399898.

[20] Kim J, Criaud M, Cho PSP, Díez-Cirarda M, Mihaescu A, Coakeley S, Ghadery C, Valli M, Jacobs MF, Houle S, Strafella AP. Abnormal intrinsic brain functional network dynamics in Parkinson's disease. *Brain.* 2017 Nov 1;140(11):2955-2967. doi: 10.1093/brain/awx233. PMID: 29053835; PMCID: PMC5841202.

[21] Zhu H, Huang J, Deng L, He N, Cheng L, Shu P, Yan F, Tong S, Sun J, Ling H. Abnormal Dynamic Functional Connectivity Associated With Subcortical Networks in Parkinson's Disease: A Temporal Variability Perspective. *Front Neurosci.* 2019 Feb 19;13:80. doi: 10.3389/fnins.2019.00080. PMID: 30837825; PMCID: PMC 6389716.

[22] Díez-Cirarda M, Strafella AP, Kim J, Peña J, Ojeda N, Cabrera-Zubizarreta A, Ibarretxe-Bilbao N. Dynamic functional connectivity in Parkinson's disease patients with mild cognitive impairment and normal cognition. *Neuroimage Clin.* 2017 Dec 9;17:847-855. doi: 10.1016/j.nicl.2017.12.013. PMID: 29527489; PMCID: PMC5842729.

[23] Peraza LR, Nesbitt D, Lawson RA, Duncan GW, Yarnall AJ, Khoo TK, Kaiser M, Firbank MJ, O'Brien JT, Barker RA, Brooks DJ, Burn DJ, Taylor JP. Intra- and inter-network functional alterations in Parkinson's disease with mild cognitive impairment. *Hum Brain*

Mapp. 2017 Mar;38(3):1702-1715. doi: 10.1002/hbm.23499. Epub 2017 Jan 13. PMID: 28084651; PMCID: PMC6866883.

[24] Klobušiaková P, Mareček R, Fousek J, Výtvarová E, Rektorová I. Connectivity Between Brain Networks Dynamically Reflects Cognitive Status of Parkinson's Disease: A Longitudinal Study. *J Alzheimers Dis.* 2019;67(3):971-984. doi: 10.3233/JAD-180834. PMID: 30776007; PMCID: PMC6398554.

[25] Vergara VM, Mayer AR, Kiehl KA, Calhoun VD. Dynamic functional network connectivity discriminates mild traumatic brain injury through machine learning. *Neuroimage Clin.* 2018 Mar 15;19:30-37. doi: 10.1016/j.nicl.2018.03.017. PMID: 30034999; PMCID: PMC6051314.

[26] Vergara VM, Mayer AR, Damaraju E, Calhoun VD. The effect of preprocessing in dynamic functional network connectivity used to classify mild traumatic brain injury. *Brain Behav.* 2017 Sep 15;7(10):e00809. doi: 10.1002/brb3.809. PMID: 29075569; PMCID: PMC5651393.

[27] Sendi MSE, Zendehrouh E, Miller RL, Fu Z, Du Y, Liu J, Mormino EC, Salat DH, Calhoun VD. Alzheimer's Disease Projection From Normal to Mild Dementia Reflected in Functional Network Connectivity: A Longitudinal Study. *Front Neural Circuits.* 2021 Jan 21;14:593263. doi: 10.3389/fncir.2020.593263. PMID: 33551754; PMCID: PMC7859281.

[28] Fu Z, Caprihan A, Chen J, Du Y, Adair JC, Sui J, Rosenberg GA, Calhoun VD. Altered static and dynamic functional network connectivity in Alzheimer's disease and subcortical ischemic vascular disease: shared and specific brain connectivity abnormalities. *Hum Brain Mapp.* 2019 Aug 1;40(11):3203-3221. doi: 10.1002/hbm.24591. Epub 2019 Apr 5. PMID: 30950567; PMCID: PMC6865624.

[29] Miller RL, Yaesoubi M, Calhoun VD. Cross-Frequency rs-fMRI Network Connectivity Patterns Manifest Differently for Schizophrenia Patients and Healthy Controls. *IEEE Signal Process*

Lett. 2016 Aug;23(8):1076-1080. doi: 10.1109/LSP.2016.2585182. PMID: 28018124; PMCID: PMC5175483.

[30] Espinoza FA, Vergara VM, Damaraju E, Henke KG, Faghiri A, Turner JA, Belger AA, Ford JM, McEwen SC, Mathalon DH, Mueller BA, Potkin SG, Preda A, Vaidya JG, van Erp TGM, Calhoun VD. Characterizing Whole Brain Temporal Variation of Functional Connectivity via Zero and First Order Derivatives of Sliding Window Correlations. *Front Neurosci.* 2019 Jun 27;13:634. doi: 10.3389/fnins.2019.00634. PMID: 31316333; PMCID: PMC6611425.

[31] Hjelm RD, Damaraju E, Cho K, Laufs H, Plis SM, Calhoun VD. Spatio-Temporal Dynamics of Intrinsic Networks in Functional Magnetic Imaging Data Using Recurrent Neural Networks. *Front Neurosci.* 2018 Sep 20;12:600. doi: 10.3389/fnins.2018.00600. PMID: 30294250; PMCID: PMC6158311.

[32] Zhou X, Ma N, Song B, Wu Z, Liu G, Liu L, Yu L, Feng J. Optimal Organization of Functional Connectivity Networks for Segregation and Integration With Large-Scale Critical Dynamics in Human Brains. *Front Comput Neurosci.* 2021 Mar 31;15:641335. doi: 10.3389/fncom.2021.641335. PMID: 33867963; PMCID: PMC 8044315.

[33] Cohen JR, D'Esposito M. The Segregation and Integration of Distinct Brain Networks and Their Relationship to Cognition. *J Neurosci.* 2016 Nov 30;36(48):12083-12094. doi: 10.1523/JNEUROSCI.2965-15.2016. PMID: 27903719; PMCID: PMC 5148214.

[34] Zhou Z, Cai B, Zhang G, Zhang A, Calhoun VD, Wang YP. Prediction and classification of sleep quality based on phase synchronization related whole-brain dynamic connectivity using resting state fMRI. *Neuroimage.* 2020 Nov 1;221:117190. doi: 10.1016/j.neuroimage.2020.117190. Epub 2020 Jul 22. PMID: 32711063.

[35] Fu Z, Iraji A, Turner JA, Sui J, Miller R, Pearlson GD, Calhoun VD. Dynamic state with covarying brain activity-connectivity: On the pathophysiology of schizophrenia. *Neuroimage.* 2021 Jan 1;224:

117385. doi: 10.1016/j.neuroimage.2020.117385. Epub 2020 Sep 17. PMID: 32950691; PMCID: PMC7781150.

[36] Calhoun VD, Kiehl KA, Pearlson GD. Modulation of temporally coherent brain networks estimated using ICA at rest and during cognitive tasks. *Hum Brain Mapp.* 2008 Jul;29(7):828-38. doi: 10.1002/hbm.20581. PMID: 18438867; PMCID: PMC2649823.

[37] Ma S, Calhoun VD, Phlypo R, Adalı T. Dynamic changes of spatial functional network connectivity in healthy individuals and schizophrenia patients using independent vector analysis. *Neuroimage.* 2014 Apr 15;90:196-206. doi: 10.1016/j.neuroimage. 2013.12.063. Epub 2014 Jan 10. PMID: 24418507; PMCID: PMC5061129.

[38] Miller RL, Vergara VM, Keator DB, Calhoun VD. A Method for Intertemporal Functional-Domain Connectivity Analysis: Application to Schizophrenia Reveals Distorted Directional Information Flow. *IEEE Trans Biomed Eng.* 2016 Dec;63(12):2525-2539. doi: 10.1109/ TBME.2016.2600637. Epub 2016 Aug 16. PMID: 27541329; PMCID: PMC5737021.

[39] Calhoun VD, Adalı T. Multisubject independent component analysis of fMRI: a decade of intrinsic networks, default mode, and neurodiagnostic discovery. *IEEE Rev Biomed Eng.* 2012;5:60-73. doi: 10.1109/RBME.2012.2211076. PMID: 23231989; PMCID: PMC4433055.

[40] Zalesky A, Fornito A, Cocchi L, Gollo LL, Breakspear M. Time-resolved resting-state brain networks. *Proc Natl Acad Sci USA.* 2014 Jul 15;111(28):10341-6. doi: 10.1073/pnas.1400181111. Epub 2014 Jun 30. PMID: 24982140; PMCID: PMC4104861.

[41] Xia Y, Chen Q, Shi L, Li M, Gong W, Chen H, Qiu J. Tracking the dynamic functional connectivity structure of the human brain across the adult lifespan. *Hum Brain Mapp.* 2019 Feb 15;40(3):717-728. doi: 10.1002/hbm.24385. Epub 2018 Dec 4. PMID: 30515914; PMCID: PMC6865727.

[42] Zhou Y, Han S. Neural dynamics of pain expression processing: Alpha-band synchronization to same-race pain but desynchronization

to other-race pain. *Neuroimage.* 2021 Jan 1;224:117400. doi: 10.1016/j.neuroimage.2020.117400. Epub 2020 Sep 24. PMID: 32979524.

[43] Tao R, Fletcher PT, Gerber S, Whitaker RT. A variational image-based approach to the correction of susceptibility artifacts in the alignment of diffusion weighted and structural MRI. *Inf Process Med Imaging.* 2009;21:664-75. doi: 10.1007/978-3-642-02498-6_55. PMID: 19694302; PMCID: PMC4031680.

[44] Zhou Y, Rodgers ZB, Kuo AH. Cerebrovascular reactivity measured with arterial spin labeling and blood oxygen level dependent techniques. *Magn Reson Imaging.* 2015 Jun;33(5):566-76. doi: 10.1016/j.mri.2015.02.018. Epub 2015 Feb 20. PMID: 25708263; PMCID: PMC4426232.

[45] Ya J, Zhou D, Ding J, Ding Y, Ji X, Yang Q, Meng R. High-resolution combined arterial spin labeling MR for identifying cerebral arterial stenosis induced by moyamoya disease or atherosclerosis. *Ann Transl Med.* 2020 Feb;8(4):87. doi: 10.21037/atm.2019.12.140. PMID: 32175380; PMCID: PMC7049068.

[46] Liang L, Lei Y, Su J, Zhou P, Lv H, Wang T, Ma T. Perfusion Quantification using Arterial Spin Labeling Magnetic Resonance Imaging after Revascularization for Moyamoya Disease. *Annu Int Conf IEEE Eng Med Biol Soc.* 2019 Jul;2019:4326-4329. doi: 10.1109/EMBC.2019.8857824. PMID: 31946825.

[47] Ha JY, Choi YH, Lee S, Cho YJ, Cheon JE, Kim IO, Kim WS. Arterial Spin Labeling MRI for Quantitative Assessment of Cerebral Perfusion Before and After Cerebral Revascularization in Children with Moyamoya Disease. *Korean J Radiol.* 2019 Jun;20(6):985-996. doi: 10.3348/kjr.2018.0651. PMID: 31132824; PMCID: PMC 6536794.

[48] Luningham JM, McArtor DB, Hendriks AM, van Beijsterveldt CEM, Lichtenstein P, Lundström S, Larsson H, Bartels M, Boomsma DI, Lubke GH. Data Integration Methods for Phenotype Harmonization in Multi-Cohort Genome-Wide Association Studies With Behavioral

Outcomes. *Front Genet.* 2019 Dec 10;10:1227. doi: 10.3389/fgene.2019.01227. PMID: 31921287; PMCID: PMC6914843.

[49] Griffith LE, van den Heuvel E, Raina P, Fortier I, Sohel N, Hofer SM, Payette H, Wolfson C, Belleville S, Kenny M, Doiron D. Comparison of Standardization Methods for the Harmonization of Phenotype Data: An Application to Cognitive Measures. *Am J Epidemiol.* 2016 Nov 15;184(10):770-778. doi: 10.1093/aje/kww098. PMID: 27769990; PMCID: PMC5141949.

[50] Clark CM, Pontecorvo MJ, Beach TG, Bedell BJ, Coleman RE, Doraiswamy PM, Fleisher AS, Reiman EM, Sabbagh MN, Sadowsky CH, Schneider JA, Arora A, Carpenter AP, Flitter ML, Joshi AD, Krautkramer MJ, Lu M, Mintun MA, Skovronsky DM; AV-45-A16 Study Group. Cerebral PET with florbetapir compared with neuropathology at autopsy for detection of neuritic amyloid-β plaques: a prospective cohort study. *Lancet Neurol.* 2012 Aug;11(8): 669-78. doi: 10.1016/S1474-4422(12)70142-4. Epub 2012 Jun 28. Erratum in: Lancet Neurol. 2012 Aug;11(8):658. PMID: 22749065.

[51] Joshi AD, Pontecorvo MJ, Lu M, Skovronsky DM, Mintun MA, Devous MD Sr. A Semiautomated Method for Quantification of F 18 Florbetapir PET Images. *J Nucl Med.* 2015 Nov;56(11):1736-41. doi: 10.2967/jnumed.114.153494. Epub 2015 Sep 3. PMID: 26338898.

[52] Manjón JV, Coupé P. volBrain: An Online MRI Brain Volumetry System. *Front Neuroinform.* 2016 Jul 27;10:30. doi: 10.3389/fninf.2016.00030. PMID: 27512372; PMCID: PMC4961698.

[53] Hutchison RM, Womelsdorf T, Allen EA, Bandettini PA, Calhoun VD, Corbetta M, Della Penna S, Duyn JH, Glover GH, Gonzalez-Castillo J, Handwerker DA, Keilholz S, Kiviniemi V, Leopold DA, de Pasquale F, Sporns O, Walter M, Chang C. Dynamic functional connectivity: promise, issues, and interpretations. *Neuroimage.* 2013 Oct 15;80:360-78. doi: 10.1016/j.neuroimage.2013.05.079. Epub 2013 May 24. PMID: 23707587; PMCID: PMC3807588.

[54] Denkova E, Nomi JS, Uddin LQ, Jha AP. Dynamic brain network configurations during rest and an attention task with frequent occurrence of mind wandering. *Hum Brain Mapp.* 2019 Oct 15;40

(15):4564-4576. doi: 10.1002/hbm.24721. Epub 2019 Aug 4. PMID: 31379120; PMCID: PMC6865814.re.

[55] Vergara VM, Miller R, Calhoun V. An information theory framework for dynamic functional domain connectivity. *J Neurosci Methods.* 2017 Jun 1;284:103-111. doi: 10.1016/j.jneumeth.2017.04. 009. Epub 2017 Apr 23. PMID: 28442296; PMCID: PMC5553686.

[56] Huang Z, Wang Q, Zhou S, Tang C, Yi F, Nie J. Exploring functional brain activity in neonates: A resting-state fMRI study. *Dev Cogn Neurosci.* 2020 Oct;45:100850. doi: 10.1016/j.dcn.2020. 100850. Epub 2020 Aug 27. PMID: 32882651; PMCID: PMC 7474406.

[57] Fu Z, Tu Y, Di X, Du Y, Pearlson GD, Turner JA, Biswal BB, Zhang Z, Calhoun VD. Characterizing dynamic amplitude of low-frequency fluctuation and its relationship with dynamic functional connectivity: An application to schizophrenia. *Neuroimage.* 2018 Oct 15;180(Pt B):619-631. doi: 10.1016/j.neuroimage.2017.09.035. Epub 2017 Sep 20. PMID: 28939432; PMCID: PMC5860934.

[58] Necka EA, Lee IS, Kucyi A, Cheng JC, Yu Q, Atlas LY. Applications of dynamic functional connectivity to pain and its modulation. *Pain Rep.* 2019 Aug 7;4(4):e752. doi: 10.1097/PR9. 0000000000000752. PMID: 31579848; PMCID: PMC6728009.

[59] Bonkhoff AK, Schirmer MD, Bretzner M, Etherton M, Donahue K, Tuozzo C, Nardin M, Giese AK, Wu O, D Calhoun V, Grefkes C, Rost NS. Abnormal dynamic functional connectivity is linked to recovery after acute ischemic stroke. *Hum Brain Mapp.* 2021 May;42(7):2278-2291. doi: 10.1002/hbm.25366. Epub 2021 Mar 2. PMID: 33650754; PMCID: PMC8046120.

[60] Espinoza FA, Anderson NE, Vergara VM, Harenski CL, Decety J, Rachakonda S, Damaraju E, Koenigs M, Kosson DS, Harenski K, Calhoun VD, Kiehl KA. Resting-state fMRI dynamic functional network connectivity and associations with psychopathy traits. *Neuroimage Clin.* 2019;24:101970. doi: 10.1016/j.nicl.2019.101970. Epub 2019 Aug 5. PMID: 31473543; PMCID: PMC6728837.

[61] Espinoza FA, Liu J, Ciarochi J, Turner JA, Vergara VM, Caprihan A, Misiura M, Johnson HJ, Long JD, Bockholt JH, Paulsen JS, Calhoun VD. Dynamic functional network connectivity in Huntington's disease and its associations with motor and cognitive measures. *Hum Brain Mapp*. 2019 Apr 15;40(6):1955-1968. doi: 10.1002/hbm.24504. Epub 2019 Jan 7. PMID: 30618191; PMCID: PMC6865767.

[62] Zhi D, Calhoun VD, Lv L, Ma X, Ke Q, Fu Z, Du Y, Yang Y, Yang X, Pan M, Qi S, Jiang R, Yu Q, Sui J. Aberrant Dynamic Functional Network Connectivity and Graph Properties in Major Depressive Disorder. *Front Psychiatry*. 2018 Jul 31;9:339. doi: 10.3389/fpsyt.2018.00339. PMID: 30108526; PMCID: PMC6080590.

Chapter 4

TYPICAL IMAGING BIOMARKERS IN SCHIZOPHRENIA AND EPILEPSY

ABSTRACT

Imaging abnormalities in schizophrenia and epilepsy had been reported with several imaging metrics previously, systematic and integrative analyses based on imaging findings are needed for better diseases diagnosis and treatment. The purposes of this chapter are to: 1. apply the relatively new dynamic functional network connectivity (dFNC) and regional homogeneity (ReHo) analyses to both schizophrenia and epilepsy patients; 2. reveal the conventional imaging differences in these two patient cohorts compared to controls with VBM, VMHC, fALFF, ReHo, ICA-DR and small-worldness methods; and 3. investigate further the commons and differences of two diseases based on comprehensive imaging findings.

Regarding the results of dFNC, reversal patterns in each state of both patient cohorts with less overall dynamics compared to controls were demonstrated. The general inter-network hypo-connectivity pattern with reduced numbers of transitions, less dwell time in majorities of states with a dip plateau form were present in epilepsy compared to schizophrenia. Conventional imaging results demonstrated significant gray matter atrophy, VMHC deficits, lower regional homogeneity pattern, static intra- and inter- network dysconnectivities as well as lower fALFF activities with different regional weighting and significance levels in two patient cohorts. Our results utilizing both conventional and relatively novel methods were in agreement with previous work, providing reliable and systematic, voxel-wise and network-based, static and dynamic, unique and multiparametric perspectives for revealing the underlying disease mechanism with accurate specifications.

Keywords: schizophrenia, epilepsy, seizure, positive and negative syndrome scale, auditory hallucination, independent vector analysis, Markov modeling, regional homogeneity, dual regression, independent component analysis, voxel-mirrored homotopic correlation, interhemispheric conductivity, efficiency, functional connectivity, brain atrophy, voxel-based morphometry, functional activity, resting-state functional connectivity, fractional amplitude of low frequency fluctuation, commons and differences

1. INTRODUCTION

Schizophrenia is a neuropsychiatric disorder with relapsed psychosis and primary symptoms of hallucination and delusion. Utilizing independent vector analysis and Markov modeling to quantify the dynamic changes of functional connectivity in schizophrenia, significantly larger fluctuations with more variable patterns of spatial concordance between frontoparietal, cerebellum and temporal lobe regions in patients were reported [1]. Also based on dynamic functional network connectivity (dFNC) analysis, patients were found to spend more time in weakly-connected states but less time in strongly-connected and activated brain states, with fractional occupancy linking to attentional performance [2]. Furthermore, these relatively weaker connectivity strengths were mainly present in the inter-subsystem, such as impaired interaction among default mode network (DMN) subsystems including posterior cingulate cortex and anterior medial prefrontal cortex hubs, in addition to the thalamocortical dysfunction in schizophrenia [2, 3]. Complementary to static functional connectivity findings including lower temporal-frontal/parietal/visual connections, less segregated motor/sensory and cognitive functions (e.g., lower task-modulation of orbitofrontal–posterior DMN and medial temporal-frontal loops) were observed when engaged with the auditory oddball task [4]. Inter-regional dependence study also revealed lower connectivity of right anterior insula but higher DMN and central executive network (CEN) connections in patients, and both were dynamically associated and related to hallucinations [5]. Finally, due to different time scale and spatiotemporal dynamics, fMRI and Magnetoencephalography (MEG) might provide distinct and complementary between-group functional connectivity differences for more informative disease mechanism elucidation of schizophrenia utilizing integrative multi-modalities [6].

Epilepsy is a neurological disease with spontaneous and recurrent seizures caused by abnormally hyper-synchrony of neuronal activity [7]. In epilepsy animal model, based on dFNC, the average daily seizure frequency was positively correlated with percentage dwell time in states with high mean functional connectivity, high segregation and integration as well as large number of transitions between states [8]. Also the frequency was negatively correlated with percentage dwell time in states with low mean functional connectivity, low segregation and integration [8]. And the dFNC (such as dwell time) was decreased in almost all four states, with changes mostly resembling the frontoparietal network and connected cerebellar/subcortical systems; suggesting disturbed communication of the frontoparietal network with other systems in frontal lobe epilepsy patients [9]. In neocortical focal epilepsy, the dynamic changes in specific cortical brain areas (neuroplasticity) might emerge to compensate the pathological epileptiform network activity for normal brain function [10]. While in the juvenile myoclonic epilepsy patients, dorsolateral prefrontal cortex (DLPFC) dFNC had higher temporal variation and dynamic characteristics [11]. A high degree of nonlinear synchronization in epileptic network was identified during seizure compared to awake time, with the main path of epileptiform activity from searching core nodes that connected with the seizure onset zone [12]. Based on simultaneous Electroencephalogram (EEG)-fMRI experiment, hypo-connectivity between ipsilateral hippocampus and DMN was caused by the left-sided interictal epileptiform discharges that might result in cognitive impairment in temporal lobe epilepsy (TLE) together with the altered reward-emotion circuit (more of the prefrontal-limbic system) and visual network [13]. Graph-theory based small-worldness analysis with phase-space trajectories of synchronous EEG signals revealed different and consistent state in epilepsy patients, with higher local (clustering coefficient) but lower global (path length) efficiencies in patients compared to controls and increased small-worldness configuration in epilepsy [14].

Using conventional voxel-based morphometry (VBM), gray matter atrophy was found in the left middle and superior temporal gyrus in first-episode (FE) for early onset schizophrenia, and was correlated with positive symptoms measured with the positive and negative syndrome scale (PANSS) [15]. The general FE schizophrenia patients had gray matter atrophy in multiple brain regions including hippocampus, fusiform, lingual gyrus, supramarginal and temporal gyri with higher gray matter volume in the middle frontal and inferior frontal operculum gyri [16]. Gray matter atrophy in several grouped networks including thalamus, insula, anterior cingulate and postcentral gyrus had also been reported in schizophrenia [17]. Schizophrenia patients also had white matter atrophy in the cerebellum and bilateral frontoparietal region together with lower fractional anisotropy (FA) values in the corpus callosum body, posterior superior longitudinal fasciculus and uncinate fasciculus [18].

Another typical imaging metric, voxel-mirrored homotopic correlation (VMHC) was used for quantifying interhemispheric conductivity that has been effective in detecting functional and microstructural abnormalities (such as demyelination) relating to neurodegenerative and neuro-developmental diseases [19, 20]. Significant reductions of VMHC in patients for a number of regions, particularly the occipital lobe, the thalamus as well as the cerebellum were detected in schizophrenia patients, and postcentral VMHC correlated with the PANSS total scores [21]. In both complete and incomplete remission patients, VMHC was lower in the visual and sensorimotor regions compared to controls, but no difference between two patient subtypes [22]. The hyper-connectivity between thalamic medial geniculate/anteroventral nucleus and auditory cortex indicated immaturities of thalamocortical connectivity that was related to the auditory hallucination in patients [23]. Also for patients with hallucinations, higher inter-network connectivity between the salience network and associative auditory network was found, and was related to hippocampal amplitude of low frequency fluctuation (ALFF) activity [24]. Similarly, higher hippocampal ALFF was associated with both auditory and visual hallucination severity in schizophrenia [25]. The global topological properties were disrupted in patients including increased nodal centralities in frontoparietal regions with decreased temporal centralities, and local clustering coefficient was related to the negative symptoms in schizophrenia [26]. Incorporating homogeneity benchmark into dFNC framework, hypo-connectivity among subcortical circuit, DMN and CEN, but hyper-connectivity between sensory networks were found in schizophrenia patients compared to controls [27].

Precise localization of epileptic focus (EF) is important for surgical intervention, and MRI/fMRI play important role in anatomical and functional mapping of normal tissue around the lesions [28]. Simultaneous EEG-fMRI recording confirmed the spatial concordance between fMRI BOLD response and seizure onset zone, and dynamic BOLD signal could capture seizure propagation regions [29]. Based on resting-state fMRI studies, locally increased excitability in the epileptogenic regions with a mixture of both hypo- and hyper- connectivity and globally decreased inter-network connections were proposed as typical connectivity alterations in the brain [30, 31]. Decreased interhemispheric functional connectivity in the temporal lobe, with higher ipsilateral peri-EF and insular as well as surrounding subcortical regions were observed in temporal lobe epilepsy [32]. Structure and function of the thalamus and thalamocortical network had been altered and were reported in several studies, such as enhanced connections between thalamus and limbic regions during seizures compared to preseizure state [33, 34].

Functional activation studies demonstrated deactivation of DMN with mainly the posterior precuneus/cingulate region and reduction of the frontal executive control network in pediatric epilepsy [35, 36]. In the genetic generalized epilepsy animal model, higher functional connectivity was reported in several brain regions including visual, motor and thalamus areas compared to control animal at resting state [37]. Also the language network was more bilaterally connected for epilepsy patients in contrast to the higher left hemispheric pattern in controls [38]. Hyper-connectivity between right DLPFC and inferior parietal lobule/superior frontal gyrus at baseline but decreased longitudinal change of connection between DLPFC/superior frontal gyrus was identified in temporal lobe epilepsy patients, with changed entropy in several regions including the supplementary motor area [39, 40]. And finally, graph-theory based analysis revealed efficiency changes including higher local clustering coefficient but lower global efficiency and centrality/synchronizability that were potential in predicting seizure frequency and duration in epilepsy patients [41-44].

Taken together, both diseases had been studied extensively with several imaging metrics, systematic and integrative analyses are needed for better diseases diagnosis and treatment. The purposes of this chapter are to: 1. apply the relatively new dFNC analysis to both schizophrenia and epilepsy patients; 2. reveal the imaging differences in these two patient cohorts compared to controls with VBM, VMHC, fractional ALFF (fALFF), regional homogeneity (ReHo), independent component analysis-based dual-regression (ICA-DR) and small-worldness methods; and 3. investigate further the commons and differences of two diseases based on these comprehensive imaging findings.

2. METHODS

2.1. Data Acquisitions in Schizophrenia Data Cohort

Schizophrenia patients and age-matched controls were included and imaging data were downloaded after approval from the Center for Biomedical Research Excellence (COBRE) website managed at the NeuroImaging Tools & Resources Collaboratory (NITRC) database (www.nitrc.org). Participants with histories of neurological disorder, mental retardation, severe head trauma with more than 5 minutes loss of consciousness, substance abuse or dependence within the last 12 months were excluded. All subjects were screened and clinical data including the Structured Clinical Interview used for DSM Disorders (SCID) diagnostic score were also collected [45, 46].

MRI experiments were performed using the 3T MRI scanner with standardized imaging protocols. The 3D multi-echo MPRAGE (MEMPR) sequence was run with TR/TI/TE = 2530/900/[1.64, 3.5, 5.36, 7.22, 9.08] ms, flip angle = 7°, matrix size = 256 x 256 x 176, resolution = 1 x 1x 1 mm^3 for reference image used in RS-fMRI connectivity/conductivity maps, as well as for structural voxel-based morphology (VBM) analysis. For the resting-state (RS)-fMRI data acquired under relaxing condition, a standard gradient-echo EPI sequence (TR/TE = 2000/29 msec, flip angle = 80°, number of volumes = 150, spatial resolution = 3 x 3 x 4 mm^3) was utilized.

Table 1. Demographic information of subjects in two groups of the Schizophrenia data cohort including controls

Group	Age (Years)	Women n/ %	Total N	Handedness (Left) n/ %	Diagnosis Score
Control	35.8 ± 1.3	23/ 31%	74	1/ 1.4%	-
Schizophrenia	38.2 ± 1.6	14/ 19%	72	10/ 13.9%	295.4 ± 0.1

As listed in Table 1, resting-state (RS)-fMRI data from 72 schizophrenia patients (age: 38.2 ± 1.6 years, 14 women and 10 left-handed; SCID diagnostic score = 295.4 ± 0.1) and 74 controls (age: 35.8 ± 1.3 years, 23 women and 1 left-handed) were included and were processed further.

2.2. Data Acquisitions in Epilepsy Data Cohort

Four epilepsy patients were downloaded from the North Shore Surgical Epilepsy Patients center and stored at the NITRC database after approval [47, 48]. RS-fMRI data were acquired under eyes closing and staying awake condition for four epilepsy patients (age: 36.5 ± 7.3 years, 3 women and all right-handed) with seizure localized at the medial temporal lobe.

Age- and gender- matched controls were chosen from the schizophrenia project and used for statistical comparisons.

All MRI experiments were performed using the 3T MRI scanner with standardized imaging protocols as well. The 3D MPRAGE sequence was obtained with TR/TI/TE = 2500/650/30 ms, flip angle = 8°, matrix size = 256 x 256 x 180, resolution = 1 x 1x 1 mm^3 for reference image and structural VBM analysis. The RS-fMRI data was acquired under relaxing condition with a standard gradient-echo EPI sequence (TR/TE = 2000/30 msec, flip angle = 70°, number of volumes = 150, spatial resolution = 3.4 x 3.4 x 4 mm^3).

2.3. Data Processing in Two Data Cohorts

Novel dynamic dFNC connectogram and regional homogeneity (ReHo) map together with typical VMHC, ICA-DR, fALFF, and small-worldness analysis were performed to two data cohorts. The details of data processing were similar to the methods listed in previous chapters and from our recently published works [19-20, 49-50]. For instance, same six typical and important functional networks were used for dFNC analysis as in previous chapter, including default mode network (DMN), frontoparietal network (FPN), salience network (SN), motor network (MN), visual network (VN) and central executive network (CEN or EN).

Regional homogeneity (ReHo) map was generated to reflect local synchrony of spontaneous neuronal activities spatially, after preprocessing the fMRI data such as motion correction and low-pass filtering using the Analysis of Functional NeuroImages (AFNI, http://afni.nimh.nih.gov) 3dReHo command. The coefficient of concordance between time series of center and neighborhood voxel was computed (e.g., 27 voxel were used as default values including the face, edge and node-wise spatial neighbors) for each voxel of the 4D fMRI data, and Z-score was derived for voxel-wise between-group comparison and global mean statistical quantification.

The MRI and fMRI images were also processed with the in-house developed scripts to derive conventional VMHC, VBM, ICA-DR, resting-state functional connectivity (RSFC), fALFF maps and small-worldness characteristics, as described in details in previous chapters and our recent works [19, 20]. Between-group comparisons of quantitative post-processed images were performed with advanced statistical tools using AFNI package and FMRIB Software Library (FSL, http://www.fmrib.ox.ac.uk/fsl) toolbox. Graph theory based small-worldness systematic analysis was computed to the functional connectivity with MRI (fcMRI) data with correlation matrix generated from 116 seeds-based RSFC, and comparisons between patients and controls were performed.

3. RESULTS

3.1. DFNC in Schizophrenia Patients

ICA components and representative networks of schizophrenia patients and controls are illustrated in Figure 1. Representative CEN together with the DMN in both controls and schizophrenia patients were demonstrated respectively. Compared to controls, lower connectivity of CEN in the DLPFC and hypo-connectivity of DMN in the left inferior parietal lobe were observed in schizophrenia patients. Connectogram of representative states S1 and S5 in both controls and schizophrenia patients is shown in Figure 2. Hyper-connectivity between FPN and VN, FPN and SN, SN and MN, SN and CEN, CEN and DMN were found in schizophrenia compared to control groups in the S1 state. On the other hand, hypo-connectivity between DMN and SN, VN and SN, VN and CEN but hyper-connectivity between DMN and MN as well as between MN and CEN existed in the S5 state. Largely reversal dynamic inter-network functional connectivity correlations and patterns in both states including lower SN but higher CEN dFNCs were exhibited in patients in contrast to controls, suggesting anti-phase synchronization and dis-coordination among functional hubs in schizophrenia.

Figure 3 presented the dynamic functional correlation matrices of states S1 and S5 in controls and schizophrenia patients respectively. The percentage of occurrence in S1 was doubled for schizophrenia compared to controls (24% vs. 12%), but decreased to about 1/3 in state S5 in patients compared to controls (11% vs. 30%). Then Figure 4 showed the frequency and mean dell time of all six states in two groups. Patients spent less time in states 2 and 5, but more time in states 1 and 3 with higher frequency and longer dell time than controls. Both had relatively low frequency and time in states 4 and 6 compared to other states. Finally the cluster occurrence distribution along the dynamic time range of six states (S1-S6) for two groups are illustrated in Figure 5 with less overall dynamics in schizophrenia compared to controls.

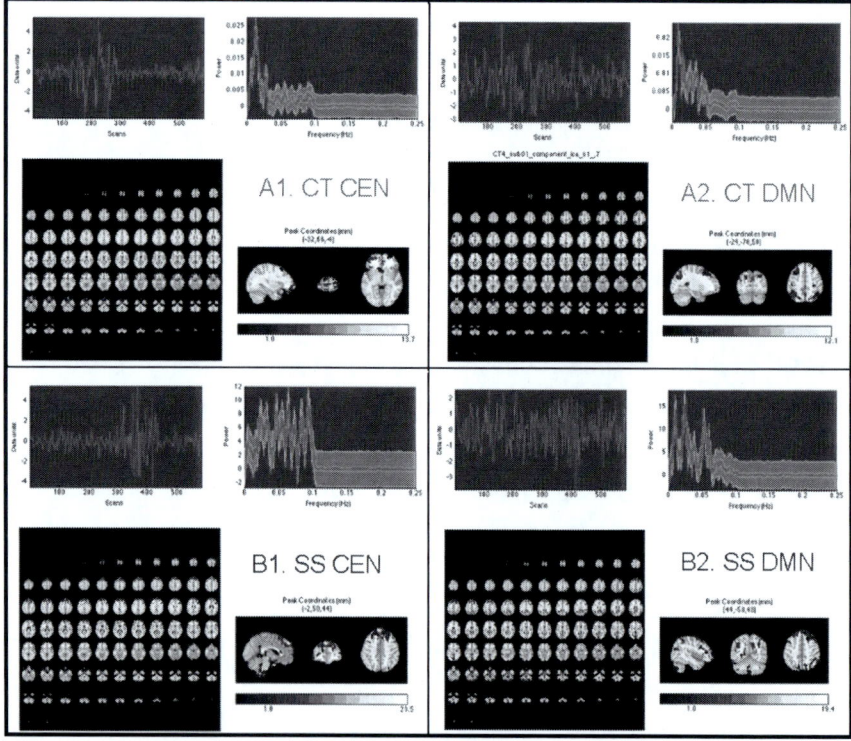

Figure 1. ICA components and representative networks. Representative central executive function (CEN) network in controls (CT) in panel A1 and schizophrenia (SS) patients in panel B1; together with the default mode network (DMN) in controls (A2) and schizophrenia (B2) respectively. Compared to controls, lower CEN in the dorsolateral prefrontal region and DMN connectivity patterns in the left inferior parietal were illustrated in schizophrenia patients.

Typical Imaging Biomarkers in Schizophrenia and Epilepsy 109

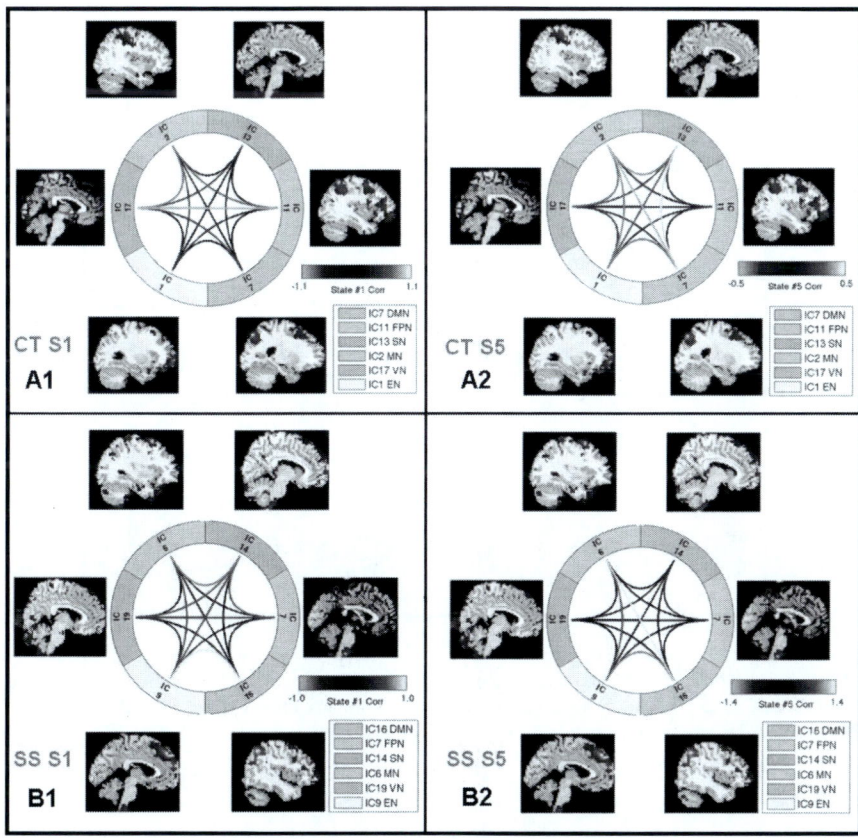

Figure 2. Connectogram of representative states S1 and S5 in control (panel A1 and A2) and schizophrenia patients (panel B1 and B2). Dynamic hyper-connectivity between FPN and VN, FPN and SN, as well as between SN and MN, SN and CEN, EN and DMN were found in schizophrenia (SS) compared to control (CT) groups in the S1 state. Hypo-connectivity between DMN and SN, FPN and SN, VN and CEN but hyper-connectivity between DMN and MN as well as between MN and CEN existed in the S5 state. Largely reversal dynamic inter-network functional connectivity correlations were found in patients in contrast to controls, suggesting anti-phase synchronization and dis-coordination in schizophrenia. Generally, lower SN but higher CEN dFNCs in schizophrenia compared to controls existed.

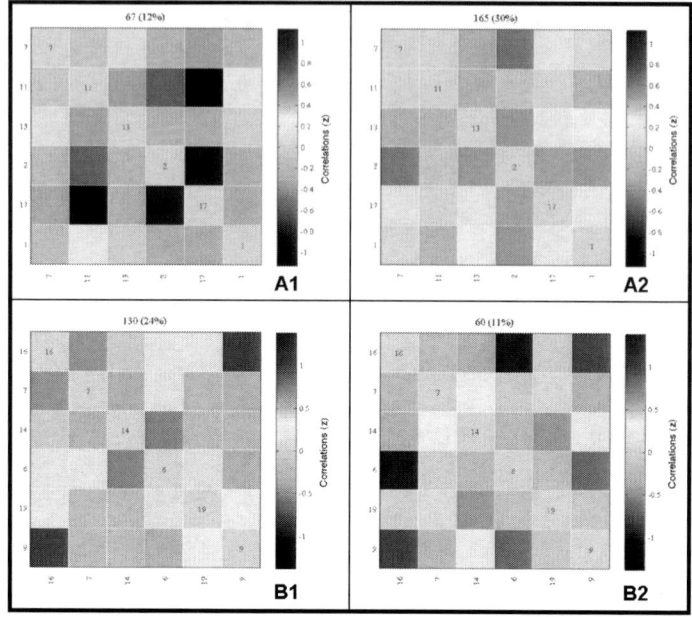

Figure 3. Dynamic functional correlation matrices of states S1 and S5 in controls (panel A1 and A2) and schizophrenia (SS) patients (panel B1 and B2) respectively. The percentage of occurrence for state S1 was doubled in schizophrenia compared to controls (24% vs. 12%), but decreased to about 1/3 for state S5 in patients compared to controls (11% vs. 30%).

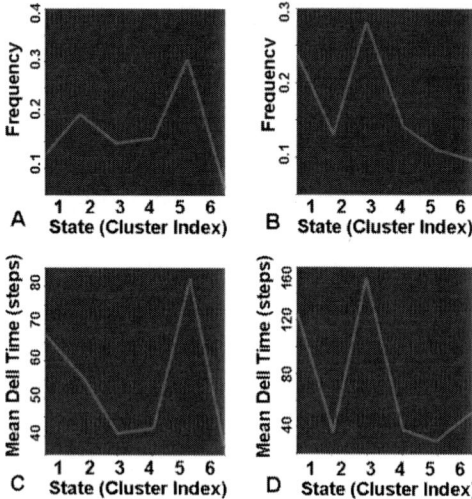

Figure 4. Frequency and mean dell time in controls (left panel - A and C respectively) as well as in schizophrenia patients (right panel - B and D). Patients spent less time in states 2 and 5, but more time in states 1 and 3 (higher frequency and longer dell time) than controls. Both had relatively low frequency and dwell time in states 4 and 6 compared to other states.

Typical Imaging Biomarkers in Schizophrenia and Epilepsy 111

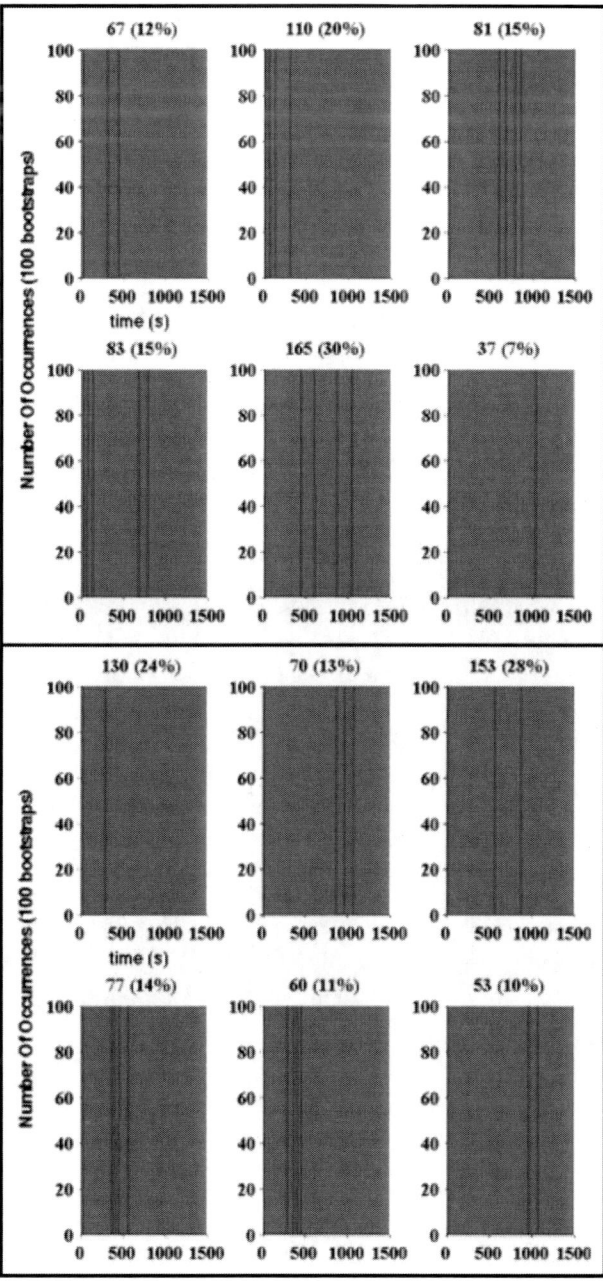

Figure 5. Cluster occurrence distribution along the dynamic time range of six states (S1-S6) in controls (upper panel) and patients (lower panel), with less overall dynamics in schizophrenia patients present.

3.2. Typical Imaging Results in Schizophrenia Patients

Typical imaging including VBM, VMHC, ReHo, fALFF and small-worldness results in schizophrenia and controls were presented in Figures 6-12. Figure 6 showed gray matter density changes in patients compared to controls with VBM (P < 0.01). Gray matter atrophy in the temporal cortex including hippocampus, middle and superior segments as well as occipitotemporal conjunction, frontal cortex including orbito- and dorso-lateral segments, insula, motor area, small ventromedial thalamic area, anterior cingulate and superior parietal lobe were found in schizophrenia patients compared to controls. On the other hand, small clusters in the medial frontal cortex showed slightly higher gray matter density in patients compared to controls (both P < 0.01).

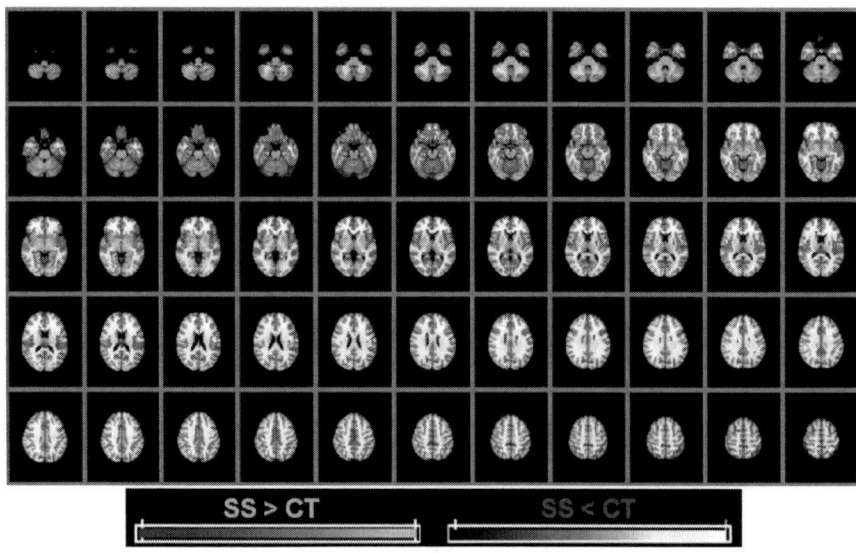

Figure 6. VBM showing gray matter density changes in patients (P < 0.01). Gray matter atrophy (red color) in the temporal cortex including hippocampus, middle and superior segments as well as occipitotemporal conjunction, frontal cortex including ventromedial, orbito- and dorso-lateral segments, insula, motor area, small ventromedial thalamic area, anterior cingulate and superior parietal lobe were found in schizophrenia (SS) patients compared to controls (CT). On the other hand, small regions in the medial frontal cortex (blue color) showed slightly higher gray matter density in patients than controls (both P < 0.01).

Figure 7 revealed the VMHC differences between two groups (P < 0.05). Higher interhemispheric correlation in the superior frontal region including DLPFC, anterior temporal, motor area, cerebellum, caudate and small regions in the posterior thalamus were found in schizophrenia patients compared to controls (P < 0.05). However, slightly lower VMHC in the anterior thalamus, superior temporal, cuneus/calcarine and postcentral/parietal opercular regions were also identified in schizophrenia compared to control participants (P < 0.05).

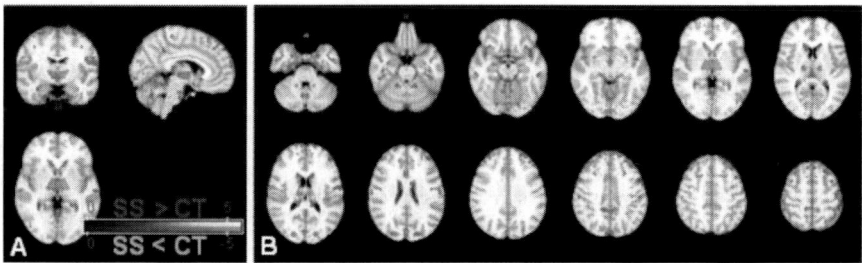

Figure 7. VMHC differences between schizophrenia (SS) patients and controls (CT). (P < 0.05). Higher interhemispheric correlations in the superior frontal including dorsolateral prefrontal cortex (DLPFC), anterior temporal, motor area, cerebellum, caudate and small regions in the posterior thalamus were found in the schizophrenia patients compared to controls (red color, P < 0.05). Slightly lower VMHC in the anterior thalamus, superior temporal, cuneus/calcarine and postcentral/parietal opercula regions were also identified in schizophrenia compared to control participants (blue, P < 0.05).

ReHo map for controls and difference between controls and schizophrenia patients are illustrated in Figure 8. Lower regional homogeneity value in the frontal, visual, parietal and superior temporal lobes were found in schizophrenia, indicating lower synchrony in patients in these regions. Slightly higher homogeneity existed in inferior temporal and white matter areas. Figure 9 showed global mean value comparisons of ReHo and fALFF, with significantly lower mean fALFF at conventional band and slow wave bands of S4 and S5 in schizophrenia patients compared to controls (P < 0.001 for conventional fALFF low frequency and S4 sub-bands, while P < 0.05 for S5 sub-band). A trend of lower global mean ReHo value existed in patients compared to controls as well (P=0.10).

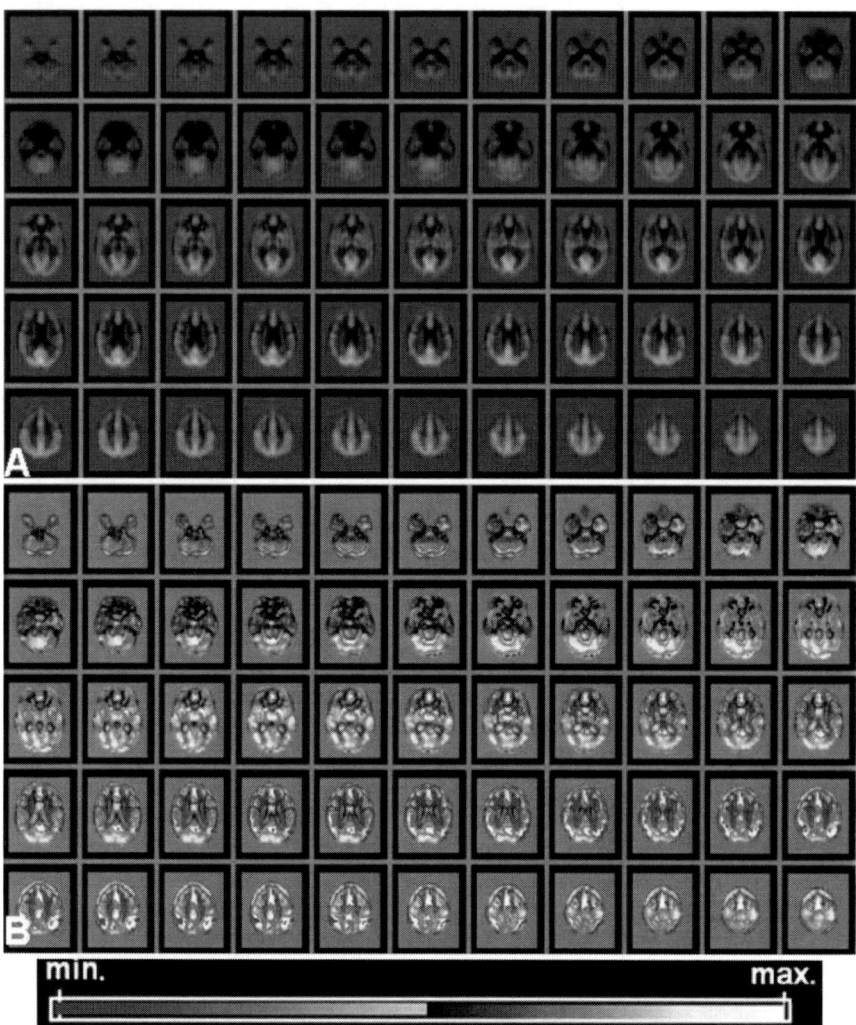

Figure 8. Regional homogeneity (ReHo) map for controls (A) and group mean difference between controls and schizophrenia patients (B). A: relatively higher ReHo in visual cortex and cortical gray matter in controls. B: Lower regional homogeneity values in schizophrenia patients compared to controls (positive red color) in the frontal, visual, parietal and superior temporal lobes were found, with slightly higher homogeneity in inferior temporal and white matter areas (negative blue color).

Typical Imaging Biomarkers in Schizophrenia and Epilepsy 115

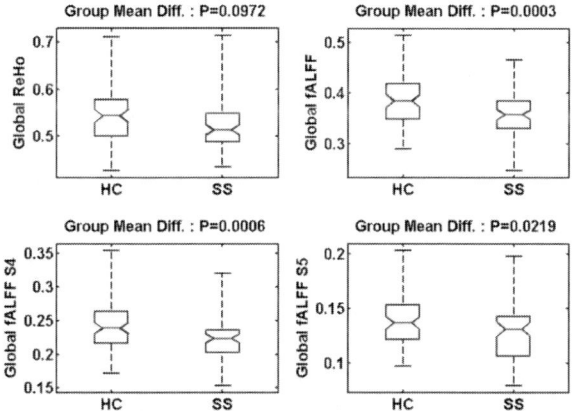

Figure 9. Global mean differences of ReHo and fALFF with significant lower fALFF at conventional and slow wave bands of S4 and S5 in schizophrenia patients compared to controls (P < 0.001 for conventional and S4 sub-bands, P < 0.05 for sub-band S5 for global fALFF).

Graph-theory based small-worldness analysis demonstrated lower global efficiency (both relative and absolute values) in schizophrenia patients compared to controls (Figure 10), together with higher local efficiency (both relative and absolute) and larger small-worldness factor (Sigma) in schizophrenia. The mean absolute global efficiency (path length) was significantly lower in patients compared to controls (P = 0.03).

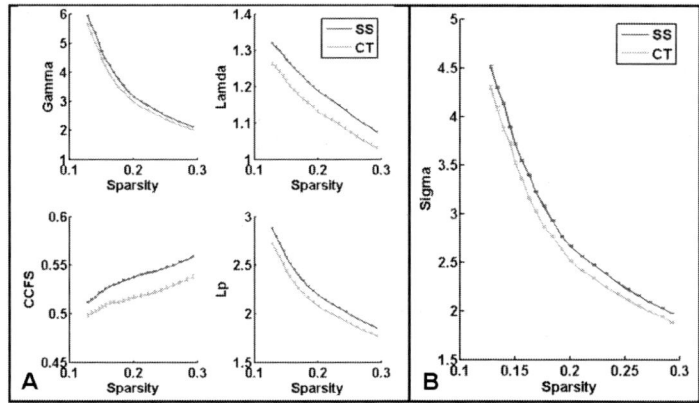

Figure 10. Graph-theory based small-worldness analysis demonstrated lower global efficiency (A: both relative Lamda and absolute Lp) in schizophrenia (SS) patients compared to controls (CT), but higher local efficiency (A: both relative and absolute, Gamma and CCFS) and larger small-worldness factor (Sigma, in B) in schizophrenia.

Gray matter density-based VBM atrophy results in schizophrenia group compared to controls were confirmed in another data cohort using voxel-wise intensity-based SPM analysis of atrophy in schizophrenia group compared to controls (P < 0.001, Figure 11). Volume atrophy in the basal ganglia, caudate, thalamus, superior temporal gyrus, scattered visual clusters, anterior cingulate, dorsolateral frontal cortex and motor area, white matter, internal capsule and minor forceps was observed in schizophrenia patients compared to controls. Furthermore, as illustrated in Figure 12, ROI-based quantification identified significantly lower regional voxel number (volume atrophy) in three brain regions in schizophrenia compared to controls (P < 0.01), including left thalamus, left and right-hemispheric white matter area.

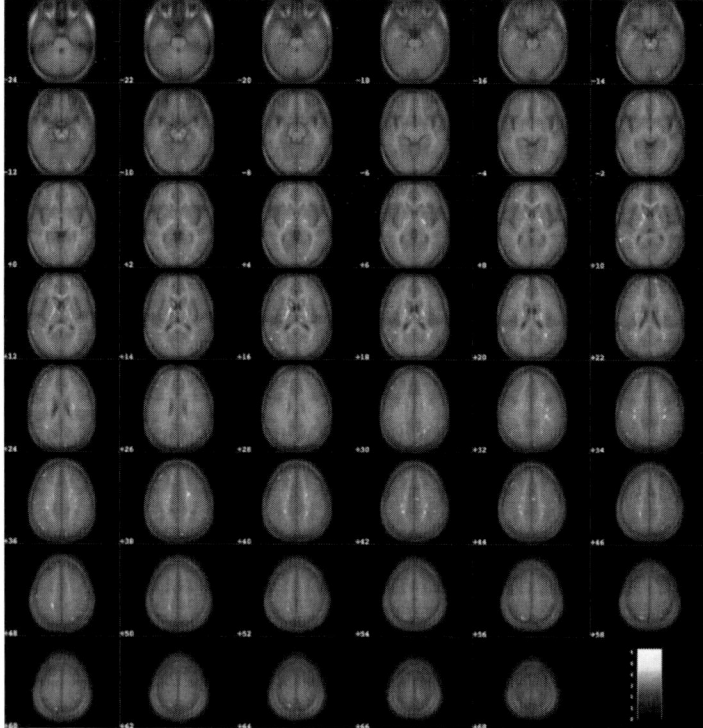

Figure 11. Voxel-wise SPM results of atrophy in schizophrenia group compared to controls (P < 0.001) after intensity normalization. Volume atrophy in the basal ganglia, caudate, thalamus, superior temporal gyrus, scattered visual clusters, anterior cingulate, dorsolateral frontal cortex and motor area, white matter cingulum, internal capsule and minor forceps was observed in schizophrenia patients compared to controls.

Typical Imaging Biomarkers in Schizophrenia and Epilepsy 117

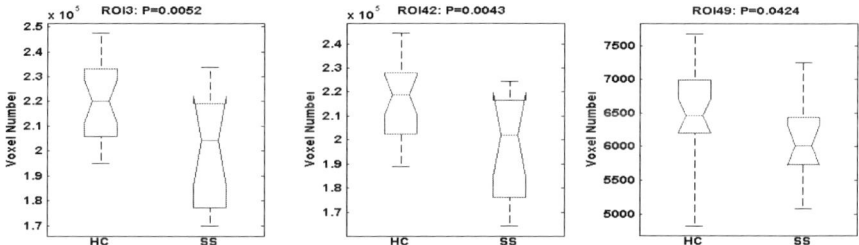

Figure 12. Significantly lower regional voxel number (atrophy) in three brain regions in schizophrenia compared to controls (P < 0.01) were identified. ROI numbers are listed as: 3- Right hemispheric white matter; 42- Left hemispheric white matter; 49- Left thalamus.

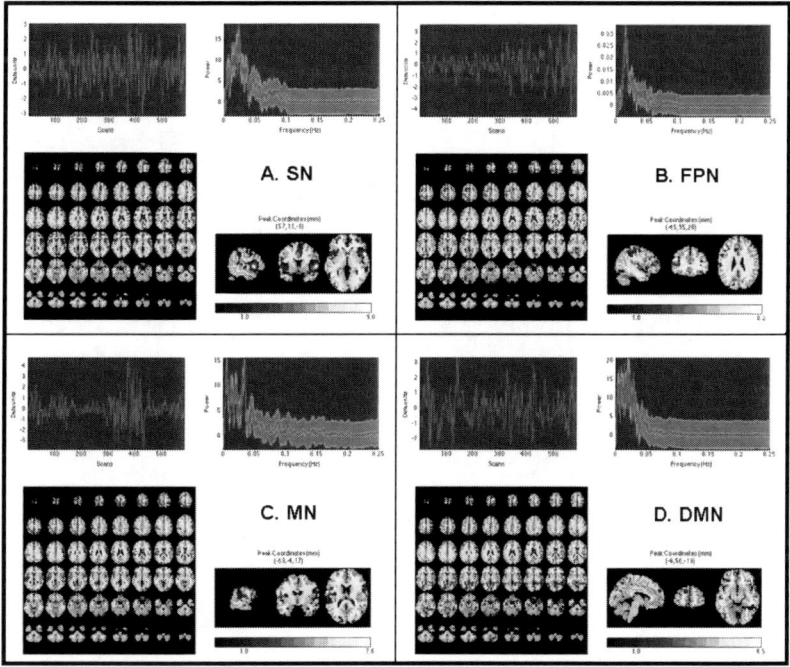

Figure 13. Time course, spectrum and spatial maps of four representative functional networks in epilepsy patients, including SN (A), FPN (B), MN (C) and DMN (D) at resting state situation. Slightly disrupted DMN pattern was observed in patients.

3.3. DFNC in Epilepsy

Time course, spectrum and spatial maps of four representative functional networks in epilepsy patients are illustrated in Figure 13, including SN, FPN, MN and DMN (Figure 13 A-D respectively) at resting state situation. Slightly disrupted DMN and FPN connectivity patterns were present in epilepsy patients. Connectogram of representative states S2 and S6 in controls and epilepsy patients are displayed in Figure 14. At state S2, the inter-network correlations of epilepsy patients were almost reversal in comparison to controls (Figure 14; A1 and B1), such as between SN and CEN(EN), SN and MN, SN and FPN, VN and CEN. At state S6, several inter-network correlations were reversal including between SN and MN, DMN and CEN, SN and CEN, FPN and CEN, FPN and VN, MN and VN.

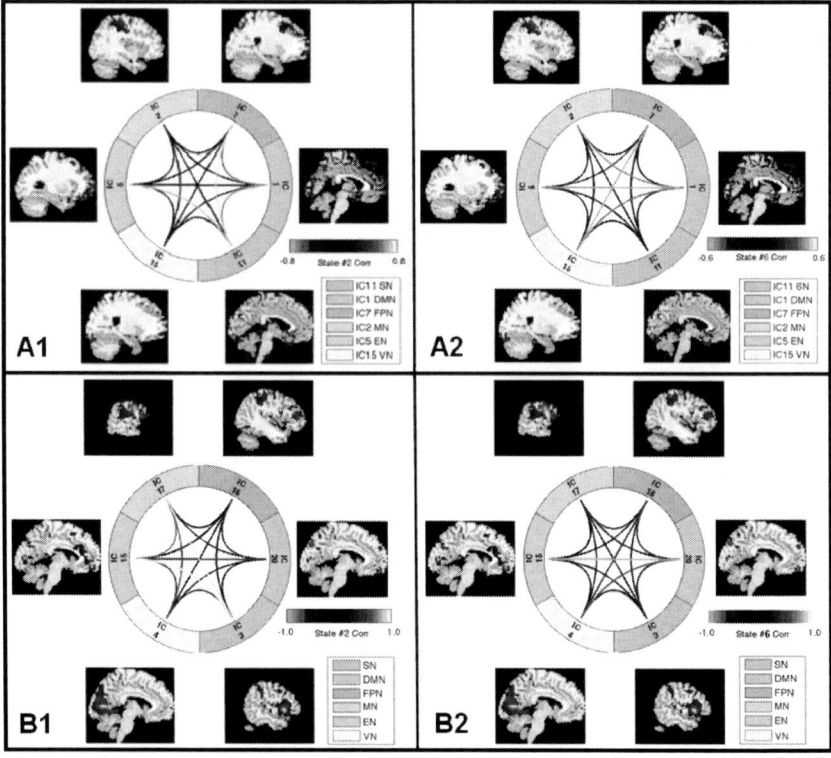

Figure 14. Connectogram of representative states S2 and S6 in controls (panel A1 and A2) and epilepsy patients (panel B1 and B2). At state S2, the inter-network correlations of epilepsy patients were almost reversal in comparison to controls (A1 and B1), such as between SN and CEN (EN), SN and MN, SN and FPN, VN and CEN, DMN and CEN, DMN and MN, DMN and VN. At state S6, several inter-network correlations were reversal including between SN and MN, DMN and CEN, DMN and MN, SN and CEN, FPN and CEN, FPN and VN, MN and VN (A2 and B2). Generally, lower DMN but higher MN connectivities in both states were found in epilepsy patients.

Typical Imaging Biomarkers in Schizophrenia and Epilepsy   119

Figure 15 showed the dFNC correlation matrices of states S2 and S6 in controls and schizophrenia patients respectively. The percentage of occurrence in S2 was much lower in patients compared to controls (5% in vs. 38%), but increased at state S6 in epilepsy (27% in patients vs. 8% in controls). Figure 16 demonstrated the occurrence, frequency and dwell time in controls and epilepsy patients. Compared to controls, patients had less evenly distributed occurrences (more focused in states 1, 5 and 6), with higher frequency and dwell time in states 1 and 5 but much less in states 2-4 compared to controls; indicating loss of dynamics in epilepsy.

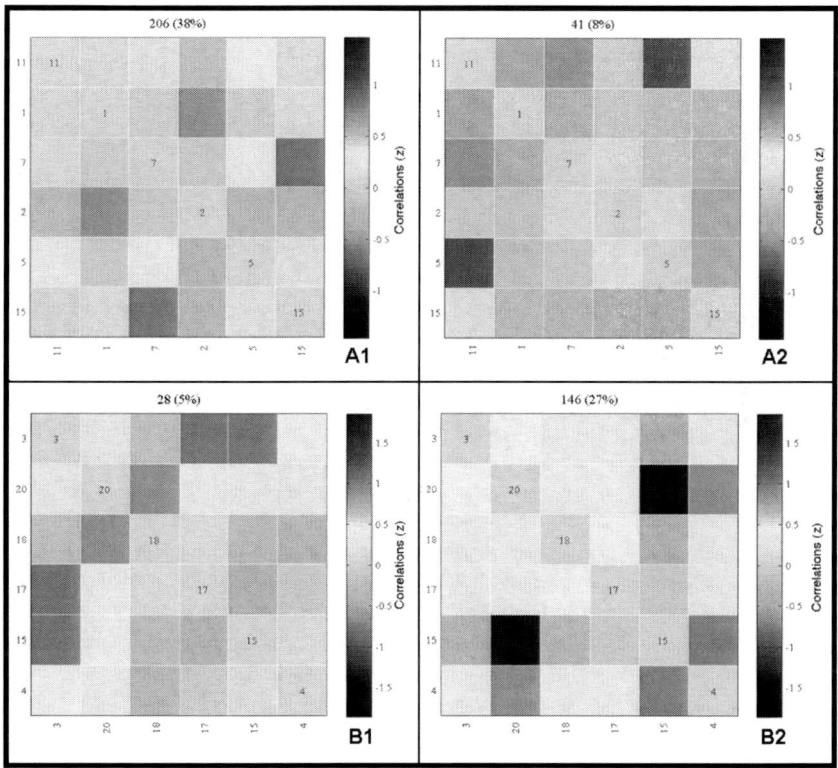

Figure 15. Dynamic functional network connectivity (dFNC) correlation matrix of states S2 and S6 in control (panel A1 and A2) and epilepsy patients (panel B1 and B2) respectively. The percentage of occurrence in S2 was much lower in patients compared to controls (5% in vs. 38%), but increased at state S6 in epilepsy (27% in patients vs. 8% in controls).

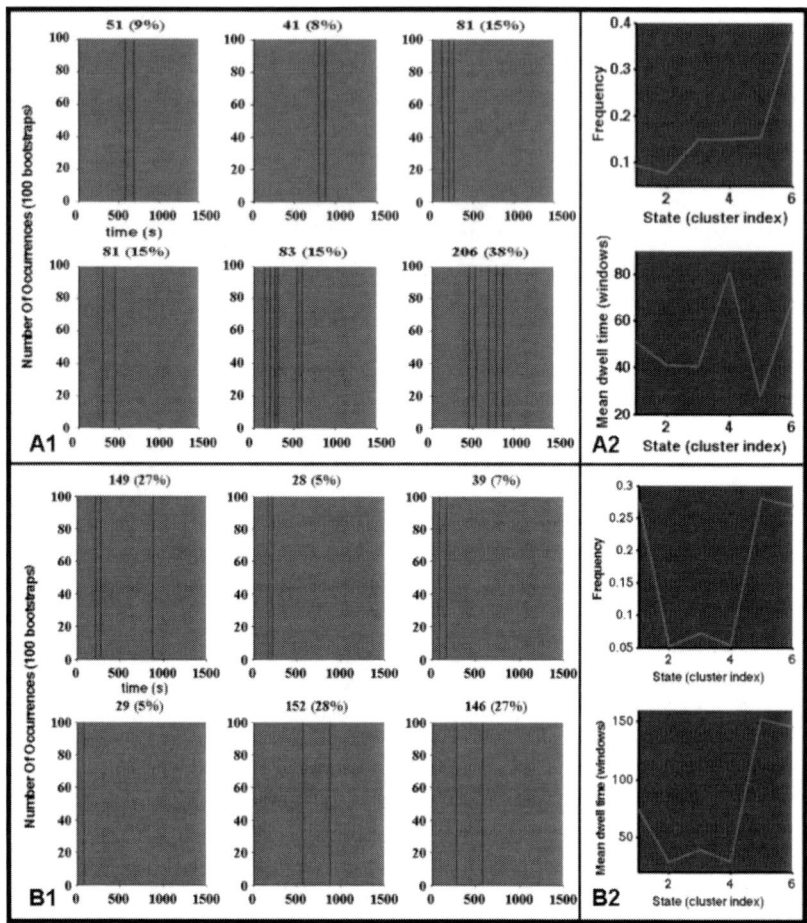

Figure 16. Occurrence (A1), frequency and dwell time (A2) in controls and epilepsy patients (B1 and B2 respectively). Compared to controls, patients had less evenly distributed occurrences (more focused in states 1, 5 and 6). Higher frequency and longer dwell time in states 1 and 5 but much less in states 2-4 were found in epilepsy compared to controls, indicating loss of dynamics in epilepsy.

3.4. Typical Imaging Application in Epilepsy

Based on the ICA-DR algorithm for intra- and inter- network remapping, decreased frontal and temporal inter-network connectivity, inter- dorso-attentional network (DAN) and DMN, intra-frontal but increased motor/supplementary motor area, inter striato-visual, thalamocortical network connectivities were illustrated in patients compared to controls (Figure 17, P < 0.001). VMHC difference between epilepsy and controls (P < 0.001) are visualized in Figure 18. Lower interhemispheric correlations in large areas of posterior visual and parietal, lateral temporal, hippocampus, orbito- and superior frontal lobes as well as cerebellum were found comparing epilepsy patients to controls. On the other hand, higher VMHC in scattered clusters in the anterior medial temporal, basal ganglia, putamen, thalamus, motor area and medial frontal regions in patients were present.

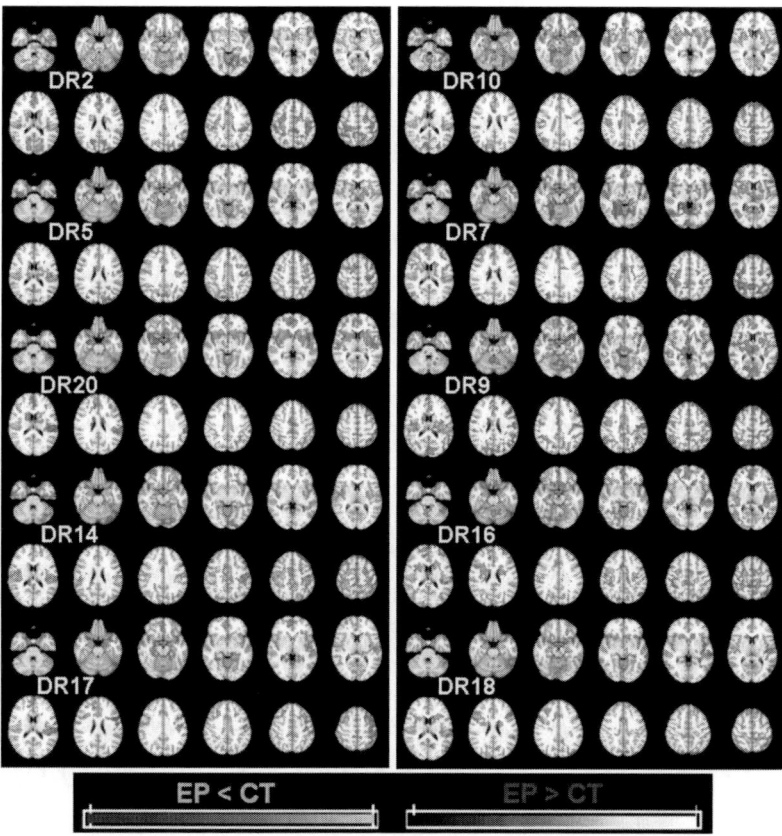

Figure 17. Based on ICA-DR algorithm, decreased frontal and temporal inter-network connectivity, inter- FPN and insular/striatum, inter- DAN and DMN, intra-frontal but increased motor/supplementary motor area, inter- striato-visual and thalamocortical network connectivities were illustrated in epilepsy patients (EP) compared to controls (CT) (P < 0.001).

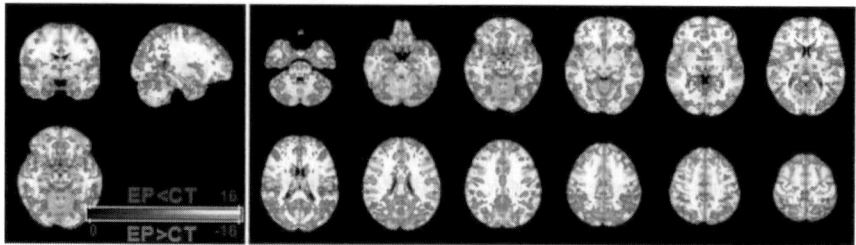

Figure 18. VMHC difference between epilepsy patients (EP) and controls (CT) with P < 0.001. Lower interhemispheric correlations in large areas of posterior visual and parietal, lateral temporal, hippocampus, orbito- and superior frontal lobes as well as cerebellum were found comparing epilepsy patients to controls (red color). Higher VMHC in scattered clusters in the anterior medial temporal, basal ganglia, putamen, thalamus, motor and supplementary motor areas and medial frontal cortex in patients existed on the other hand (blue color).

The ReHo pattern of epilepsy showed lower regional homogeneity in areas of temporal, orbito-medial prefrontal and parietal lobes in epilepsy patients (Figure 19). Lower global efficiency (both relative and absolute) in epilepsy patients compared to controls, together with slightly higher local efficiency (mainly absolute) and larger small-worldness factor were observed in epilepsy (Figure 20). The small-worldness characteristics (i.e., lower global but higher local efficiencies) in epilepsy patients in comparison to controls were similar to schizophrenia, but with a much less degree of difference.

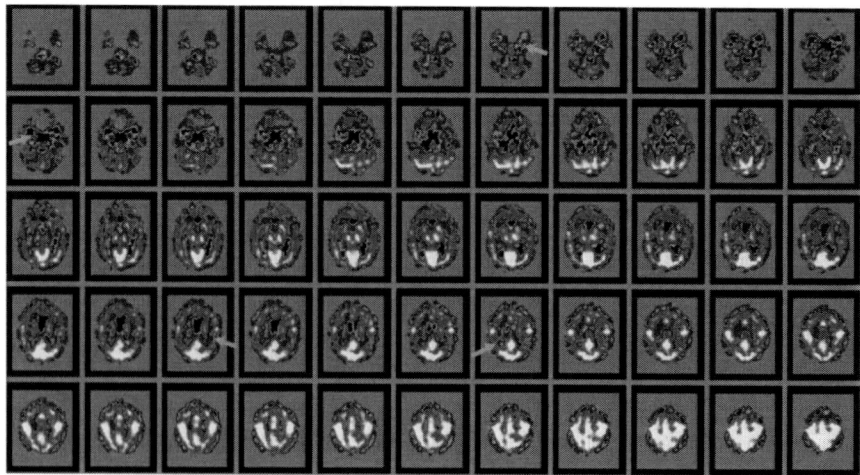

Figure 19. Group mean ReHo pattern of epilepsy showing lower regional homogeneity (blue color) in areas of temporal, orbito-medial prefrontal and parietal lobes (green arrows).

Typical Imaging Biomarkers in Schizophrenia and Epilepsy 123

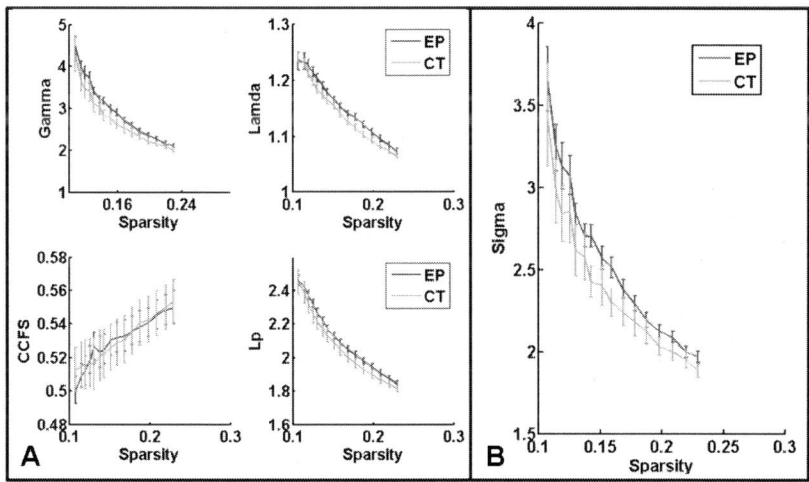

Figure 20. Slightly lower global efficiency (A: both relative Lamda and absolute Lp) in epilepsy patients (EP) compared to controls (CT), together with slightly higher local efficiency (A: absolute Gamma) and larger small-worldness factor (Sigma, in B) in epilepsy patients. The small-worldness characteristics in epilepsy were similar to schizophrenia, but with a less degree of difference.

4. DISCUSSION

4.1. Summary of Results

Based on the results of dFNC, reversal patterns of two representative states in both patient cohorts with less overall dynamics compared to controls were demonstrated. These anti-phase synchronization and dis-coordination between dynamic neuronal networks in both patients were likely due to injuries in the thalamus and dorsolateral prefrontal regions (executive control dysfunction) in schizophrenia, and thalamic-related hippocampal sclerosis or brain lesions in critical temporal lobe hubs that were in charge of brain wave generation and persistence in epilepsy [23, 32-34, 49-50]. The general inter-network hypo-connectivity pattern, showing reduced numbers of transitions and less dwell time in majorities of states with dip plateau form, was present in epilepsy compared to schizophrenia. Our results were consistent with previous dFNC findings, indicating that epilepsy patients tend to stay in more negative and static brain states, while schizophrenia tend to switch between positive and negative states and both having different brain paces or waveforms from controls [1-14].

Representative typical imaging results demonstrated significant gray matter atrophy in schizophrenia patients in regions of frontal, thalamus and visual/temporal/parietal lobes based on VBM. And large brain areas showed VMHC deficits (asynchrony or discoordination) in epilepsy patients including the posterior temporal/parietal/cerebellum regions compared to controls. Small-worldness analysis identified lower global but higher local efficiencies in both patient groups, with larger degree of differences in comparison to controls were found for schizophrenia group than epilepsy patients. Lower regional homogeneity (ReHo map) was illustrated in frontal, visual, parietal and superior temporal lobes for schizophrenia, together with lower ReHo pattern in temporal, orbito-medial prefrontal and parietal lobes for epilepsy. These observations of more frontal and visual neuronal regional asynchrony in schizophrenia in contrast to more temporal and motor affected in temporal lobe epilepsy were in line with the disease etiology of spatial specificities in two patient cohorts [15-17, 21-26]. Finally, some other imaging differences were identified as well; for instance, both intra- and inter- network dysconnectivities based on ICA-DR algorithm were found in epilepsy. These asynchronous neural network activity and connectivity in epilepsy included lower intra- frontal and temporal network connectivity, inter-FPN and insula/striatum, inter DMN and DAN connections; but no significant differences in schizophrenia. Furthermore, lower fALFF activities in S4/S5 sub-bands and general low-frequency band were found in schizophrenia but not in epilepsy patients, that might be due to more significant and larger-area local neural activity injuries in schizophrenia. Consistency remained between dFNC and conventional methods such as lower SN but higher CEN connectivities reflected from both dynamic connectogram and VMHC conductivity in schizophrenia patients, as well as lower DMN but higher MN inter-network modulations results from both dFNC and ICA-DR algorithms for epilepsy.

4.2. Schizophrenia and Epilepsy: Commons and Differences

In people with a history of epilepsy, schizophrenia risk increased (relative risk factor of 2.48) as well as the schizophrenia-like psychosis (risk factor of 2.93), including family history of psychosis and epilepsy [51]. Common structural brain abnormalities in both epilepsy and psychosis such as diffuse brain lesions (digenesis) interacted with the presentation of each other, and led to association between epilepsy and schizophrenia-like psychosis [52]. The leucine-rich glioma inactivated (LGI) family gene loci might be the shared risk gene for both diseases, especially epilepsy with regional auditory interference and schizophrenia patients with auditory hallucination [53]. Both schizophrenia and epilepsy patients had gray matter atrophy in the temporal lobe including superior temporal gyrus and frontoparietal region compared to controls, as well as an extension even beyond temporal lobe in epilepsy with psychosis [54]. Brain network dysfunction in DMN, SN, CEN and/or DAN were demonstrated in both patient groups [55]. Fronto-limbic deficits such as frontal hypoactivity and medial temporal hyperactivity with variable proportion in the "two-hit" model for schizophrenia and epilepsy-related psychosis formed the convergent basis of a systematic neurobiological model to explain the complex whole-brain network disorders [56].

Brain connectome could help elucidate the epileptic excitation, quantify seizure propagation and severity as well as localize seizure spread and territories interaction, with a possible precise brain network model for improving surgical guidance [57]. For instance, hippocampal sclerosis, cortical development abnormalities and vascular malformations were some common signs of epilepsy, and better prediction of seizure together with timely monitoring of disease progression as well as effective treatment with multiple imaging modalities are some ongoing work [58]. As another example of application, simultaneous EEG-fMRI recording allowed transient quantification and spatiotemporal dynamic monitoring of hemodynamic function during epileptic discharges as well as subsequent network modification and cognitive impact [59]. Furthermore, significant reductions of betweenness centrality, a global efficiency factor and especially the loss of central hubs in the frontal and temporal lobes were observed in schizophrenia patients with less global information integration capacity [60]. In addition, based on structural cortical thickness metric, lower global but higher local efficiencies together with lower DMN centrality but higher paralimbic nodal centrality were confirmed in schizophrenia patients compared to controls, indicating patients had suboptimal topology of brain resource utilization and organization [61]. And white matter dysconnectivity in the areas of medial frontal, parietal/occipital and left temporal lobes were also observed in schizophrenia, with up to 20% less efficiently for patients in contrast to controls [62].

4.3. Summary and Future Work

In summary, we had reported comprehensive large-scale imaging findings with conventional and relatively novel methods in both schizophrenia and epilepsy patients, including both the commons and differences of two diseases. For instance, lower DMN but higher MN dFNCs were found in epilepsy patients that were consistent with the state-dependent clinical symptom of the disease. Also lower SN but higher CEN dFNCs in schizophrenia were similar to the lower SN dFNC results for CBS/PSP patients under two different resting state situations (conditional and state-shifting role of SN) in Chapter 3. Our results were in agreement with previous works, providing reliable and systematic, voxel-wise and network-based, static and dynamic, unique and multiparametric perspectives for revealing the underlying disease mechanism with accurate specifications.

Some future works include combination of other imaging modalities such as simultaneous EEG-fMRI and PET/MRI for better spatiotemporal neuronal source localization and microscopic confirmation with molecular underpins as well as connections to behavioral and neurocognitive metrics. Generalization of our methods to larger data cohorts with more participants and validation with well-designed state-specific/condition-dependent disease models together with physiological experiments will be another future goal [63]. The unique and combined, novel and conventional imaging features utilized in this book that could pinpoint the exact abnormalities of several atypical diseases provided illustrative and confirmative results as application cases of cutting-edge and advanced imaging methods in special and challenging brain disorders.

ACKNOWLEDGMENTS

The schizophrenia and epilepsy imaging data used in this chapter were obtained from the multi-center Functional Connecome Project (http://fcon_1000.projects.nitrc.org). And we would like to thank NITRC center for storage of the original data, especially the INDI Retrospective Data Sharing Samples. In accordance with HIPAA guidelines and 1000 functional Connectomes Project/INDI protocols, all datasets were de-identified and approved for usage.

REFERENCES

[1] Ma S, Calhoun VD, Phlypo R, Adalı T. Dynamic changes of spatial functional network connectivity in healthy individuals and schizophrenia patients using independent vector analysis. *Neuroimage.* 2014 Apr 15;90:196-206. doi: 10.1016/j.neuroimage. 2013.12.063. Epub 2014 Jan 10. PMID: 24418507; PMCID: PMC 5061129.

[2] Fu Z, Iraji A, Turner JA, Sui J, Miller R, Pearlson GD, Calhoun VD. Dynamic state with covarying brain activity-connectivity: On the pathophysiology of schizophrenia. *Neuroimage.* 2021 Jan 1;224: 117385. doi: 10.1016/j.neuroimage.2020.117385. Epub 2020 Sep 17. PMID: 32950691; PMCID: PMC7781150.

[3] Du Y, Pearlson GD, Yu Q, He H, Lin D, Sui J, Wu L, Calhoun VD. Interaction among subsystems within default mode network diminished in schizophrenia patients: A dynamic connectivity approach. *Schizophr Res.* 2016 Jan;170(1):55-65. doi: 10.1016/j.schres.2015.11.021. Epub 2015 Dec 3. PMID: 26654933; PMCID: PMC4707124.

[4] Sakoğlu U, Pearlson GD, Kiehl KA, Wang YM, Michael AM, Calhoun VD. A method for evaluating dynamic functional network connectivity and task-modulation: application to schizophrenia. *MAGMA.* 2010 Dec;23(5-6):351-66. doi: 10.1007/s10334-010-0197-8. Epub 2010 Feb 17. PMID: 20162320; PMCID: PMC2891285.

[5] Manoliu A, Riedl V, Zherdin A, Mühlau M, Schwerthöffer D, Scherr M, Peters H, Zimmer C, Förstl H, Bäuml J, Wohlschläger AM, Sorg C. Aberrant dependence of default mode/central executive network interactions on anterior insular salience network activity in schizophrenia. *Schizophr Bull.* 2014 Mar;40(2):428-37. doi: 10.1093/schbul/sbt037. Epub 2013 Mar 21. PMID: 23519021; PMCID: PMC3932085.

[6] Sanfratello L, Houck JM, Calhoun VD. Dynamic Functional Network Connectivity in Schizophrenia with Magnetoencephalography and Functional Magnetic Resonance Imaging: Do Different Timescales Tell a Different Story? *Brain Connect.* 2019 Apr;9(3):251-262. doi: 10.1089/brain.2018.0608. PMID: 30632385; PMCID: PMC6479258.

[7] Wurina, Zang YF, Zhao SG. Resting-state fMRI studies in epilepsy. *Neurosci Bull.* 2012 Aug;28(4):449-55. doi: 10.1007/s12264-012-1255-1. PMID: 22833042; PMCID: PMC5561896.

[8] Christiaen E, Goossens MG, Descamps B, Larsen LE, Boon P, Raedt R, Vanhove C. Dynamic functional connectivity and graph theory metrics in a rat model of temporal lobe epilepsy reveal a preference for brain states with a lower functional connectivity, segregation and integration. *Neurobiol Dis.* 2020 Jun;139:104808. doi: 10.1016/j.nbd.2020.104808. Epub 2020 Feb 19. PMID: 32087287.

[9] Klugah-Brown B, Luo C, He H, Jiang S, Armah GK, Wu Y, Li J, Yin W, Yao D. Altered Dynamic Functional Network Connectivity in Frontal Lobe Epilepsy. *Brain Topogr.* 2019 May;32(3):394-404. doi: 10.1007/s10548-018-0678-z. Epub 2018 Sep 25. PMID: 30255350.

[10] Pedersen M, Omidvarnia A, Curwood EK, Walz JM, Rayner G, Jackson GD. The dynamics of functional connectivity in neocortical focal epilepsy. *Neuroimage Clin.* 2017 Apr 11;15:209-214. doi: 10.1016/j.nicl.2017.04.005. PMID: 28529877; PMCID: PMC 5429237.

[11] Wang Y, Berglund IS, Uppman M, Li TQ. Juvenile myoclonic epilepsy has hyper dynamic functional connectivity in the dorsolateral frontal cortex. *Neuroimage Clin.* 2019;21:101604. doi: 10.1016/j.nicl.2018.11.014. Epub 2018 Nov 19. PMID: 30527355; PMCID: PMC6412974.

[12] Mei T, Wei X, Chen Z, Tian X, Dong N, Li D, Zhou Y. Epileptic foci localization based on mapping the synchronization of dynamic brain network. *BMC Med Inform Decis Mak.* 2019 Jan 31;19(Suppl 1):19. doi: 10.1186/s12911-019-0737-8. PMID: 30700279; PMCID: PMC 6354332.

[13] Tong X, An D, Xiao F, Lei D, Niu R, Li W, Ren J, Liu W, Tang Y, Zhang L, Zhou B, Gong Q, Zhou D. Real-time effects of interictal spikes on hippocampus and amygdala functional connectivity in unilateral temporal lobe epilepsy: An EEG-fMRI study. *Epilepsia.* 2019 Feb;60(2):246-254. doi: 10.1111/epi.14646. Epub 2019 Jan 17. PMID: 30653664.

[14] Lang P, Liu DB, Cai SM, Hong L, Zhou PL. Recurrence network analysis of the synchronous EEG time series in normal and epileptic brains. *Cell Biochem Biophys.* 2013 Jun;66(2):331-6. doi: 10.1007/s12013-012-9452-0. PMID: 23090787.

[15] Tang J, Liao Y, Zhou B, Tan C, Liu W, Wang D, Liu T, Hao W, Tan L, Chen X. Decrease in temporal gyrus gray matter volume in first-episode, early onset schizophrenia: an MRI study. *PLoS One.* 2012;7(7):e40247. doi: 10.1371/journal.pone.0040247. Epub 2012 Jul 3. PMID: 22802957; PMCID: PMC3388989.

[16] Chang M, Womer FY, Bai C, Zhou Q, Wei S, Jiang X, Geng H, Zhou Y, Tang Y, Wang F. Voxel-Based Morphometry in Individuals at Genetic High Risk for Schizophrenia and Patients with Schizophrenia during Their First Episode of Psychosis. *PLoS One.* 2016 Oct 10;11(10):e0163749. doi: 10.1371/journal.pone.0163749. Erratum in: *PLoS One.* 2017 Jan 9;12 (1):e0170146. PMID: 27723806; PMCID: PMC5056757.

[17] Glahn DC, Laird AR, Ellison-Wright I, Thelen SM, Robinson JL, Lancaster JL, Bullmore E, Fox PT. Meta-analysis of gray matter anomalies in schizophrenia: application of anatomic likelihood estimation and network analysis. *Biol Psychiatry.* 2008 Nov 1;64(9):774-81. doi: 10.1016/j.biopsych.2008.03.031. Epub 2008 May 16. PMID: 18486104; PMCID: PMC5441233.

[18] Lei W, Li N, Deng W, Li M, Huang C, Ma X, Wang Q, Guo W, Li Y, Jiang L, Zhou Y, Hu X, McAlonan GM, Li T. White matter alterations in first episode treatment-naïve patients with deficit schizophrenia: a combined VBM and DTI study. *Sci Rep.* 2015 Aug 10;5:12994. doi: 10.1038/srep12994. PMID: 26257373; PMCID: PMC4530339.

[19] Zhou Y. *Joint Imaging Applications in General Neurodegenerative Disease: Parkinson's, Frontotemporal, Vascular Dementia and Autism.* Nova Science Publishers. 2021.

[20] Zhou Y. *Imaging and Multiomic Biomarker Applications: Advances in Early Alzheimer's Disease.* Nova Science Publishers. 2021.

[21] Hoptman MJ, Zuo XN, D'Angelo D, Mauro CJ, Butler PD, Milham MP, Javitt DC. Decreased interhemispheric coordination in schizophrenia: a resting state fMRI study. *Schizophr Res.* 2012 Oct;141(1):1-7. doi: 10.1016/j.schres.2012.07.027. Epub 2012 Aug 19. PMID: 22910401; PMCID: PMC3446206.

[22] Lang X, Wang L, Zhuo CJ, Jia F, Wang LN, Wang CL. Reduction of Interhemispheric Functional Connectivity in Sensorimotor and Visual Information Processing Pathways in Schizophrenia. *Chin Med J (Engl).* 2016 Oct 20;129(20):2422-2426. doi: 10.4103/0366-6999.191758. PMID: 27748333; PMCID: PMC5072253.

[23] Mancini V, Zöller D, Schneider M, Schaer M, Eliez S. Abnormal Development and Dysconnectivity of Distinct Thalamic Nuclei in Patients With 22q11.2 Deletion Syndrome Experiencing Auditory Hallucinations. *Biol Psychiatry Cogn Neurosci Neuroimaging*. 2020 Sep;5(9):875-890. doi: 10.1016/j.bpsc.2020.04.015. Epub 2020 May 8. PMID: 32620531.

[24] Hare SM, Law AS, Ford JM, Mathalon DH, Ahmadi A, Damaraju E, Bustillo J, Belger A, Lee HJ, Mueller BA, Lim KO, Brown GG, Preda A, van Erp TGM, Potkin SG, Calhoun VD, Turner JA. Disrupted network cross talk, hippocampal dysfunction and hallucinations in schizophrenia. *Schizophr Res*. 2018 Sep;199:226-234. doi: 10.1016/j.schres.2018.03.004. Epub 2018 Mar 21. PMID: 29571753; PMCID: PMC6148405.

[25] Hare SM, Ford JM, Ahmadi A, Damaraju E, Belger A, Bustillo J, Lee HJ, Mathalon DH, Mueller BA, Preda A, van Erp TG, Potkin SG, Calhoun VD, Turner JA; Functional Imaging Biomedical Informatics Research Network. Modality-Dependent Impact of Hallucinations on Low-Frequency Fluctuations in Schizophrenia. *Schizophr Bull*. 2017 Mar 1;43(2):389-396. doi: 10.1093/schbul/sbw093. PMID: 27421792; PMCID: PMC5605256.

[26] Jiang Y, Yao D, Zhou J, Tan Y, Huang H, Wang M, Chang X, Duan M, Luo C. Characteristics of disrupted topological organization in white matter functional connectome in schizophrenia. *Psychol Med*. 2020 Sep 3:1-11. doi: 10.1017/S0033291720003141. Epub ahead of print. PMID: 32880241.

[27] Rahaman MA, Damaraju E, Turner JA, van Erp T, Mathalon DH, Vaidya J, Mueller BA, Pearlson G, Calhoun V. Tri-clustering dynamic functional network connectivity (dFNC) identifies significant schizophrenia effects across multiple states in distinct subgroups of individuals. *Brain Connect*. 2021 May 28. doi: 10.1089/brain.2020.0896. Epub ahead of print. PMID: 34049447.

[28] Seiler A, Nöth U, Hok P, Reiländer A, Maiworm M, Baudrexel S, Meuth S, Rosenow F, Steinmetz H, Wagner M, Hattingen E, Deichmann R, Gracien RM. Multiparametric Quantitative MRI in

Neurological Diseases. *Front Neurol.* 2021 Mar 8;12:640239. doi: 10.3389/fneur.2021.640239. PMID: 33763021; PMCID: PMC 7982527.

[29] Wang J, Jing B, Liu R, Li D, Wang W, Wang J, Lei J, Xing Y, Yan J, Loh HH, Lu G, Yang X. Characterizing the seizure onset zone and epileptic network using EEG-fMRI in a rat seizure model. *Neuroimage.* 2021 May 2;237:118133. doi: 10.1016/j.neuroimage. 2021.118133. Epub ahead of print. PMID: 33951515.

[30] Luo C, Qiu C, Guo Z, Fang J, Li Q, Lei X, Xia Y, Lai Y, Gong Q, Zhou D, Yao D. Disrupted functional brain connectivity in partial epilepsy: a resting-state fMRI study. *PLoS One.* 2011;7(1):e28196. doi: 10.1371/journal.pone.0028196. Epub 2012 Jan 5. PMID: 22242146; PMCID: PMC3252302.

[31] Courtiol J, Guye M, Bartolomei F, Petkoski S, Jirsa VK. Dynamical Mechanisms of Interictal Resting-State Functional Connectivity in Epilepsy. *J Neurosci.* 2020 Jul 15;40(29):5572-5588. doi: 10.1523/JNEUROSCI.0905-19.2020. Epub 2020 Jun 8. PMID: 32513827; PMCID: PMC7363471.

[32] Maccotta L, He BJ, Snyder AZ, Eisenman LN, Benzinger TL, Ances BM, Corbetta M, Hogan RE. Impaired and facilitated functional networks in temporal lobe epilepsy. *Neuroimage Clin.* 2013 Jun 25;2:862-72. doi: 10.1016/j.nicl.2013.06.011. PMID: 24073391; PMCID: PMC3777845.

[33] Peng SJ, Hsin YL. Altered structural and functional thalamo-cortical networks in secondarily generalized extratemporal lobe seizures. *Neuroimage Clin.* 2016 Nov 12;13:55-61. doi: 10.1016/j.nicl. 2016.11.010. PMID: 27942447; PMCID: PMC5133650.

[34] Yan Y, Xie G, Zhou H, Liu H, Wan M. Altered spontaneous brain activity in patients with childhood absence epilepsy: associations with treatment effects. *Neuroreport.* 2020 May 22;31(8):613-618. doi: 10.1097/WNR.0000000000001447. PMID: 32366812.

[35] Oyegbile TO, VanMeter JW, Motamedi GK, Bell WL, Gaillard WD, Hermann BP. Default mode network deactivation in pediatric temporal lobe epilepsy: Relationship to a working memory task and

executive function tests. *Epilepsy Behav.* 2019 May;94:124-130. doi: 10.1016/j.yebeh.2019.02.031. Epub 2019 Mar 22. PMID: 30909075; PMCID: PMC7333914.

[36] Oyegbile TO, VanMeter JW, Motamedi G, Zecavati N, Santos C, Chun CLE, Gaillard WD, Hermann B. Executive dysfunction is associated with an altered executive control network in pediatric temporal lobe epilepsy. *Epilepsy Behav.* 2018 Sep;86:145-152. doi: 10.1016/j.yebeh.2018.04.022. Epub 2018 Jul 9. PMID: 30001910; PMCID: PMC7395827.

[37] Salinas FS, Szabó CÁ. Resting-state functional connectivity in the baboon model of genetic generalized epilepsy. *Epilepsia.* 2015 Oct;56(10):1580-9. doi: 10.1111/epi.13115. Epub 2015 Aug 20. PMID: 26290449; PMCID: PMC4593742.

[38] Mbwana JS, You X, Ailion A, Fanto EJ, Krishnamurthy M, Sepeta LN, Newport EL, Vaidya CJ, Berl MM, Gaillard WD. Functional connectivity hemispheric contrast (FC-HC): A new metric for language mapping. *Neuroimage Clin.* 2021 Mar 1;30:102598. doi: 10.1016/j.nicl.2021.102598. Epub ahead of print. PMID: 33858809; PMCID: PMC8102641.

[39] Qin L, Jiang W, Zheng J, Zhou X, Zhang Z, Liu J. Alterations Functional Connectivity in Temporal Lobe Epilepsy and Their Relationships With Cognitive Function: A Longitudinal Resting-State fMRI Study. *Front Neurol.* 2020 Jul 21;11:625. doi: 10.3389/fneur.2020.00625. Erratum in: *Front Neurol.* 2020 Oct 27;11:614081. PMID: 32793090; PMCID: PMC7385240.

[40] Zhou M, Jiang W, Zhong D, Zheng J. Resting-state brain entropy in right temporal lobe epilepsy and its relationship with alertness. *Brain Behav.* 2019 Nov;9(11):e01446. doi: 10.1002/brb3.1446. Epub 2019 Oct 12. PMID: 31605452; PMCID: PMC6851803.

[41] Bernhardt BC, Bernasconi N, Hong SJ, Dery S, Bernasconi A. Subregional Mesiotemporal Network Topology Is Altered in Temporal Lobe Epilepsy. *Cereb Cortex.* 2016 Jul;26(7):3237-48. doi: 10.1093/cercor/bhv166. Epub 2015 Jul 28. PMID: 26223262; PMCID: PMC4898674.

[42] Hao J, Luo W, Xie Y, Feng Y, Sun W, Peng W, Zhao J, Zhang P, Ding J, Wang X. Functional Network Alterations as Markers for Predicting the Treatment Outcome of Cathodal Transcranial Direct Current Stimulation in Focal Epilepsy. *Front Hum Neurosci.* 2021 Mar 17;15:637071. doi: 10.3389/fnhum.2021.637071. PMID: 33815082; PMCID: PMC8009991.

[43] Haneef Z, Chiang S. Clinical correlates of graph theory findings in temporal lobe epilepsy. *Seizure.* 2014 Nov;23(10):809-18. doi: 10.1016/j.seizure.2014.07.004. Epub 2014 Jul 23. PMID: 25127370; PMCID: PMC4281255.

[44] van Dellen E, Douw L, Baayen JC, Heimans JJ, Ponten SC, Vandertop WP, Velis DN, Stam CJ, Reijneveld JC. Long-term effects of temporal lobe epilepsy on local neural networks: a graph theoretical analysis of corticography recordings. *PLoS One.* 2009 Nov 26;4(11):e8081. doi: 10.1371/journal.pone.0008081. PMID: 19956634; PMCID: PMC2778557.

[45] Mayer AR, Ruhl D, Merideth F, Ling J, Hanlon FM, Bustillo J, Cañive J. Functional imaging of the hemodynamic sensory gating response in schizophrenia. *Hum Brain Mapp.* 2013 Sep;34(9):2302-12. doi: 10.1002/hbm.22065. Epub 2012 Mar 28. PMID: 22461278; PMCID: PMC4020570.

[46] Stephen JM, Coffman BA, Jung RE, Bustillo JR, Aine CJ, Calhoun VD. Using joint ICA to link function and structure using MEG and DTI in schizophrenia. *Neuroimage.* 2013 Dec;83:418-30. doi: 10.1016/j.neuroimage.2013.06.038. Epub 2013 Jun 15. PMID: 23777757; PMCID: PMC3815989.

[47] Keller CJ, Bickel S, Entz L, Ulbert I, Milham MP, Kelly C, Mehta AD. Intrinsic functional architecture predicts electrically evoked responses in the human brain. *Proc Natl Acad Sci USA.* 2011 Jun 21;108(25):10308-13. doi: 10.1073/pnas.1019750108. Epub 2011 Jun 2. Erratum in: *Proc Natl Acad Sci USA.* 2011 Oct 11;108(41):17234. PMID: 21636787; PMCID: PMC3121855.

[48] Alonazi BK, Keller schizophrenia, Fallon N, Adams V, Das K, Marson AG, Sluming V. Resting-state functional brain networks in

adults with a new diagnosis of focal epilepsy. *Brain Behav.* 2019 Jan;9(1):e01168. doi: 10.1002/brb3.1168. Epub 2018 Nov 28. PMID: 30488645; PMCID: PMC6346674.

[49] Zhou Y. *Multiparametric Imaging in Neurodegenerative Disease.* Nova Science Publishers. 2019.

[50] Zhou Y. *Neuroimaging in Mild Traumatic Brain Injury.* Nova Science Publishers. 2021.

[51] Qin P, Xu H, Laursen TM, Vestergaard M, Mortensen PB. Risk for schizophrenia and schizophrenia-like psychosis among patients with epilepsy: population based cohort study. *BMJ.* 2005 Jul 2;331(7507): 23. doi: 10.1136/bmj.38488.462037.8F. Epub 2005 Jun 17. PMID: 15964859; PMCID: PMC558534.

[52] Sachdev P. Schizophrenia-like psychosis and epilepsy: the status of the association. *Am J Psychiatry.* 1998 Mar;155(3):325-36. doi: 10.1176/ajp.155.3.325. PMID: 9501741.

[53] Cascella NG, Schretlen DJ, Sawa A. Schizophrenia and epilepsy: is there a shared susceptibility? *Neurosci Res.* 2009 Apr;63(4):227-35. doi: 10.1016/j.neures.2009.01.002. PMID: 19367784; PMCID: PMC 2768382.

[54] Marsh L, Sullivan EV, Morrell M, Lim KO, Pfefferbaum A. Structural brain abnormalities in patients with schizophrenia, epilepsy, and epilepsy with chronic interictal psychosis. *Psychiatry Res.* 2001 Nov 5;108(1):1-15. doi: 10.1016/s0925-4927(01)00115-9. PMID: 11677063.

[55] Li Q, Liu S, Guo M, Yang CX, Xu Y. The Principles of Electroconvulsive Therapy Based on Correlations of Schizophrenia and Epilepsy: A View From Brain Networks. *Front Neurol.* 2019 Jun 27;10:688. doi: 10.3389/fneur.2019.00688. PMID: 31316456; PMCID: PMC6610531.

[56] Butler T, Weisholtz D, Isenberg N, Harding E, Epstein J, Stern E, Silbersweig D. Neuroimaging of frontal-limbic dysfunction in schizophrenia and epilepsy-related psychosis: toward a convergent neurobiology. *Epilepsy Behav.* 2012 Feb;23(2):113-22. doi: 10.1016/

j.yebeh.2011.11.004. Epub 2011 Dec 29. PMID: 22209327; PMCID: PMC3339259.

[57] Davis KA, Jirsa VK, Schevon CA. Wheels Within Wheels: Theory and Practice of Epileptic Networks. *Epilepsy Curr*. 2021 May 14:15357597211015663. doi: 10.1177/15357597211015663. Epub ahead of print. PMID: 33988042.

[58] Adamczyk B, Węgrzyn K, Wilczyński T, Maciarz J, Morawiec N, Adamczyk-Sowa M. The Most Common Lesions Detected by Neuroimaging as Causes of Epilepsy. *Medicina* (Kaunas). 2021 Mar 22;57(3):294. doi: 10.3390/medicina57030294. PMID: 33809843; PMCID: PMC8004256.

[59] Shamshiri EA, Sheybani L, Vulliemoz S. The Role of EEG-fMRI in Studying Cognitive Network Alterations in Epilepsy. *Front Neurol*. 2019 Sep 24;10:1033. doi: 10.3389/fneur.2019.01033. PMID: 31608007; PMCID: PMC6771300.

[60] van den Heuvel MP, Mandl RC, Stam CJ, Kahn RS, Hulshoff Pol HE. Aberrant frontal and temporal complex network structure in schizophrenia: a graph theoretical analysis. *J Neurosci*. 2010 Nov 24;30(47):15915-26. doi: 10.1523/JNEUROSCI.2874-10.2010. PMID: 21106830; PMCID: PMC6633761.

[61] Zhou Y, Chou KH, Lo CY, Su TP, Jiang T. Abnormal topological organization of structural brain networks in schizophrenia. *Schizophr Res*. 2012 Nov;141(2-3):109-18. doi: 10.1016/j.schres.2012.08.021. Epub 2012 Sep 13. PMID: 22981811.

[62] Zalesky A, Fornito A, Seal ML, Cocchi L, Westin CF, Bullmore ET, Egan GF, Pantelis C. Disrupted axonal fiber connectivity in schizophrenia. *Biol Psychiatry*. 2011 Jan 1;69(1):80-9. doi: 10.1016/j.biopsych.2010.08.022. Epub 2010 Oct 29. PMID: 21035793; PMCID: PMC4881385.

[63] Cui Y, Li M, Biswal B, Jing W, Zhou C, Liu H, Guo D, Xia Y, Yao D. Dynamic Configuration of Coactive Micropatterns in the Default Mode Network During Wakefulness and Sleep. *Brain Connect*. 2021 Apr 19. doi: 10.1089/brain.2020.0827. Epub ahead of print. PMID: 33403904.

ABOUT THE AUTHOR

Yongxia Zhou, PhD
Scientist
Departments of Biomedical Engineering and Radiology
University of Southern California

Yongxia Zhou is a medical imaging scientist specializing in neuroimaging and neuroscience applications. She had completed her PhD degree from University of Southern California in biomedical imaging in 2004 and had been trained and worked as a neuroimaging scientist in several prestigious institutes including Columbia University, New York University, University of Pennsylvania and NIH. Her research focuses on multi-modal neuroimaging including using MRI/PET and EEG instrumentation as well as their integration to make the best usage of each modality and to help interpret underlying co-existing pathophysiological mechanisms for better disease diagnosis and treatment. Her specific interests in MRI technology include brain mapping of blood flow, oxygen saturation and extraction fraction and metabolism as well as vascular reactivity assessment with fMRI activity/connectivity and arterial spin labeling (ASL)-based blood flow measures. Applications of these advanced techniques in multiple domains including memory, cognition, and neurodegenerative diseases such as dementia and brain injury are the main focus. She has published more than 14 books, 5 book chapters, and 100 papers and abstracts in well-known international journals and conferences. She has also served as editor and reviewer for several journals, books and international conferences including *JMRI*, *JCBFM*, *HBM*, *AJNR*, *PlosOne*, *ISMRM* and *ICAD*.

INDEX

#

4- repeat tauopathy neuroimaging initiative (4RTNI), 35, 36, 55

A

A4 trial, 70
abnormal, 33, 53, 54, 57, 66, 86, 91, 97, 131, 136
absolute global efficiency, 16, 18, 115
accuracy, xvi, 2, 64, 66
AD sequencing project (ADSP)- phenotype harmonization consortium (PHC), 70, 70
ADNI center, 5, 71
ADNI laboratory of neuroimaging (LONI), 36
ADSP-PHC composite scores, 70
Adult Changes in Thought (ACT), 70
aerobic exercise, 20
AFNI, 106, 107
age, 2, 6, 35, 36, 70, 71, 104, 105
age-matched, 104
aging effects, 19
alien limb, viii, 33, 55

alien limb syndrome, 33, 55
Alzheimer's disease (AD), xii, xv, xvi, 2, 3, 4, 7, 22, 33, 35, 37, 47, 49, 63, 64, 66, 67, 69, 70, 79, 81, 82, 83, 86, 90, 96, 134
amplitude of low frequency fluctuation (ALFF), xi, 7, 37, 65, 103, 104
amygdala, 42, 85, 129
amyloid, xvi, 11, 12, 19, 64, 70, 71, 84, 85, 86, 96
amyloid accumulation, 11, 12, 71, 84, 85
amyloid deposition, xvi, 64, 84, 86
amyloid imaging, 71
analysis framework, 65
anatomical MRI, 70
anatomical normalization, 6
animal model, 101, 103
anisotropy reduction, 34
anterior cingulate, ix, x, xiv, xvi, 9, 15, 17, 20, 32, 43, 44, 52, 64, 71, 84, 86, 102, 112, 116
anterior cingulate cortex, ix, xiv, 15, 20, 32, 43, 44
anterior cingulum, 33
anterior temporal lobe, ix, xiv, 3, 32, 40, 41, 42, 43, 44, 52

anterior thalamic radiation, ix, xv, 32, 37, 43, 47, 49, 53
anti-amyloid treatment, 70
antinociceptive system, 87
anti-phase synchronization, xi, 107, 109, 123
arterial spin labeling (ASL), xv, xvi, 63, 64, 69, 79, 82, 83, 86, 95, 137
ASL-CBF, xvi, 64, 86
associated spatial map, ix, 64
asymptomatic, v, xii, xv, xvi, 63, 64, 71, 84, 85, 86
asymptomatic AD, xii
asymptomatic Alzheimer's, xv, 63, 70
asymptomatic Aβ+ carriers, xvi, 64, 85, 87
asynchronous neural network activity, 124
attention, vii, 2, 3, 25, 86, 96
attention and memory deficits, 3
attentional performance, 100
atypical Parkinson's, v, viii, xii, 31, 33, 88
atypical Parkinsonism, viii, 33, 88
auditory hallucination, 100, 102, 125
auditory oddball task, 101
automatic clustering, 65
axial diffusivity (AD), xii, xv, xvi, 2, 3, 4, 7, 22, 33, 35, 37, 47, 49, 63, 64, 66, 67, 69, 70, 79, 81, 82, 83, 86, 90, 96, 134
Aβ1-42 accumulation, 20

B

band pass temporal filtering, 68
basal ganglia, viii, xiv, 8, 9, 10, 13, 15, 17, 19, 20, 31, 32, 38, 39, 40, 41, 42, 43, 44, 45, 47, 51, 52, 53, 59, 66, 116, 121, 122
basal ganglia midline, 42
baseline, 3, 11, 12, 19, 25, 66, 104
behavioral symptoms, 54
behavioral-related shifts, 65
betweenness centrality, 125
biological markers, 4, 35, 69

brain abnormalities, viii, xi, xiii, 2, 21, 125, 135
brain atrophy, vii, viii, xiii, xiv, 1, 2, 21, 31, 54, 100
brain connectome, 125
brain disorders, xii, 127
brain lesions, xi, 123
brain network dynamics, 66
brain network dysfunction, xi, 125
brain networks, vii, ix, xiii, 1, 21, 28, 64, 94, 134, 136
brain organization, x, 67
brain reserve, 20
brain resource utilization, 126
brain states, xi, 87, 100, 124, 128
brain stem, viii, 14, 32, 34, 35, 36, 38, 39, 48
brain wave generation, xi, 123

C

calcarine, 9, 38, 39, 113
caudate, 3, 9, 13, 14, 33, 38, 39, 40, 42, 113, 116
CBF quantification, 70
Center for Biomedical Research Excellence (COBRE), 104
center for imaging of neurodegenerative diseases (CIND), 69
central executive network (CEN), x, xi, xv, 63, 64, 66, 68, 71, 73, 77, 78, 86, 87, 101, 103, 106, 107, 108, 109, 118, 124, 125, 126, 128
central hubs, 126
central opercularis, 13
central operculum, 33
central sulci, 34
centrality, 33, 88, 104, 126
cerebellar reference, 71
cerebellar-insular connectivity, 34

cerebral blood flow (CBF), xii, xv, xvi, 63, 64, 69, 70, 79, 81, 82, 83, 86
cerebrospinal fluid (CSF), 3
cingulum, ix, xv, 32, 37, 43, 47, 49, 52, 53, 54, 116
cingulum connecting the hippocampus, ix, xv, 32, 47, 49, 53
cingulum of the hippocampus connection, 37
circle plot, 82, 84
classification performance, 66
clinical features, 34, 57, 60
clinical measures, 87
clinical phenotypes, 54
clinical symptoms, 33, 34, 54
clustering coefficient, 102, 103, 104
cognition improvement, 54
cognitive adaption, x, 65
cognitive decline, 3, 20, 25, 28, 29, 90
cognitive domains, vii, 2
cognitive impact, 125
cognitive impairment, 3, 20, 23, 24, 25, 54, 101
cognitive performance, 3, 88
cognitive profile, vii, 3
cognitive relevance, 65
cognitive scores, 66, 82
cognitive tests, 19, 65, 83
cognitive training, 20
commons and differences, xiii, xvi, 99, 100, 104, 126
commons and differences of imaging results, xiii
comorbid disease prevention, xiii, 2, 21
comorbid disorder, 21
compensation, viii, xiii, 1, 17, 18, 21
complexity, 25, 67
composite cognitive scores, 79, 82
composite score, xiii, xvi, 64, 70, 82, 86
composite summary, 71
comprehensive analysis, xiv, 31, 34
concurrent patterns, 65, 90

condition-dependent disease model, 127
conductivity, xi, 20, 36, 42, 105, 124
connectogram, 64, 67, 68, 69, 72, 73, 77, 78, 88, 106, 107, 109, 118, 124
conventional band, 113
conventional hubs, 5
conventional imaging, xi, xiii, xv, xvi, 63, 64, 67, 87, 99, 127
conventional imaging findings, xv, 63, 67
cornu ammonis (CA), viii, 5, 7, 65, 91, 136
corpus callosum, 3, 25, 54, 102
corpus callosum shrinkage, 54
correlation matrix, 7, 65, 69, 74, 79, 107, 119
correlational test, 64
cortical development abnormalities, 125
cortical function compensation, 53
cortical hyper-connectivity, 33
cortical motor circuits, 66
corticobasal degeneration (CBD), viii, xiv, 31, 32, 34, 43, 44, 45, 46, 53, 54, 55, 57, 58, 60, 61, 62, 64
corticobasal syndrome (CBS), v, viii, x, xi, xii, xiv, xv, 31, 32, 33, 34, 35, 36, 38, 39, 40, 41, 42, 43, 44, 45, 46, 47, 48, 49, 50, 51, 52, 53, 54, 55, 57, 58, 59, 61, 63, 67, 69, 71, 72, 73, 74, 75, 76, 77, 78, 79, 80, 81, 86, 88, 126
corticospinal tract, 33, 37, 47, 49, 53
corticostriatal, 9, 43, 44
cross domain mutual information (CDMI), 87
cuneus, 9, 11, 12, 13, 14, 38, 39, 113

D

data sharing, 65
deep gray matter structure, 33
deep sleep, 66
default mode network (DMN), vii, xi, xii, xiii, 1, 2, 3, 5, 7, 8, 9, 10, 11, 15, 16, 19,

Index

20, 21, 24, 43, 44, 45, 46, 52, 64, 66, 68, 71, 72, 73, 76, 77, 78, 87, 100, 101, 103, 106, 107, 108, 109, 117, 118, 120, 121, 124, 125, 126, 128, 132
delusion, x, 100
dementia, xi, 3, 21, 22, 23, 25, 26, 28, 54, 58, 89, 92, 130, 137
dementia onset delay, 21
demyelination, 3, 102
dentate gyrus (DG), 5, 7, 19, 62
depleted dopamine, 3
depression scale, 3
depressive symptom, 88
detection power, 65
detrending, 68
dFNC algorithm, 66, 67
diagnosis criteria, 54
diagnostic criterion, 20
diagnostic score, 105
diffuse brain lesions, xi, 125
diffusion tensor imaging (DTI), ix, x, xii, 3, 32, 35, 36, 37, 53, 86, 88, 130, 134
diffusivity, 32, 34, 37, 47, 49, 53, 54
diffusivity increase, 34
dip plateau, xi, xvi, 99, 123
dip plateau form, xi, xvi, 99, 123
disease classification, 66
disease detection, xvi, 64, 87
disease diagnosis, viii, xii, 137
disease mechanism, xii, xvii, 100, 101, 126
disease models, xii, 127
disease profile, xiii, 1, 4
disease progression, 125
disease severity, 3
disinhibition function, xv, 64, 86
disorder impairing eye movements, viii, 33
DMN sub-network risk factor, xii
donepezil treatment, 4
dorso-attentional network (DAN), viii, 5, 9, 15, 16, 19, 20, 21, 120, 121, 124, 125
dorso-lateral prefrontal cortex (DLPFC), 9, 10, 15, 16, 43, 44, 52, 101, 104, 107, 113

dorsolateral prefrontal cortex (DLPFC), 9, 10, 15, 16, 43, 44, 52, 101, 104, 107, 113
dual regression, viii, 2, 9, 32, 100
dwell time, x, xi, xvi, 64, 66, 69, 76, 87, 99, 101, 110, 119, 120, 123
dynamic BOLD signal, 103
dynamic correlation, 65, 67, 68
dynamic correlation matrix, 67
dynamic fALFF, 87
dynamic fluctuations, 65
dynamic functional connectivity, 65, 89, 90, 91, 94, 96, 97, 128, 129
dynamic functional network connectivity (dFNC), ix, xi, xii, xv, xvi, 63, 64, 65, 66, 67, 68, 69, 72, 73, 74, 77, 78, 79, 86, 87, 88, 90, 92, 97, 98, 99, 100, 101, 103, 104, 106, 119, 123, 124, 126, 128, 131
dynamic network changes, xiii
dynamic temporal correlation, 65
dynamic transitions, x, 79, 86
dynamic windows, ix, 65
dynamics, x, xv, 64, 67, 68, 74, 79, 86, 88, 89, 90, 91, 93, 94, 119, 120, 129
dystonia, viii, 33

E

early AD, vii, xiii, 1, 5, 7, 21, 70
early MCI (EMCI), xiii, 1, 2, 4, 5, 7, 8, 9, 19
early prevention, xii, 4, 20
EEG entropy, 3
EEG power spectrum, 66
effective treatment, 20, 54, 125
efficiency, 2, 32, 48, 50, 53, 56, 100, 104
efficiency changes, 104
efficient treatment, viii, xiii, 2, 21
elbow criterion, 67
electroencephalogram (EEG), 3, 25, 26, 66, 90, 102, 103, 129, 132, 136, 137
electrophysiological source, 66

entropy, 104, 133
epilepsy, v, xi, xiii, xvi, 99, 100, 101, 103, 104, 105, 117, 118, 119, 120, 121, 122, 123, 124, 125, 126, 127, 128, 129, 132, 133, 134, 135, 136
epileptic discharges, 125
epileptic excitation, 125
epileptic focus (EF), x, 103
epileptic network, 101, 132
epileptiform activity, 101
epileptiform network, 101
excitability, 103
executive control dysfunction, xi, 123
executive control network, 103, 133
executive function, vii, 2, 19, 20, 70, 79, 108, 133
eye-moving centers, viii, 33
eyes closing, xii, xiv, 32, 35, 36, 38, 64, 66, 69, 105
eyes opening, 32, 64

F

first-episode (FE), 102, 129
fMRI, x, 5, 6, 7, 16, 18, 25, 35, 36, 37, 66, 67, 68, 69, 87, 88, 90, 92, 93, 94, 97, 101, 103, 105, 106, 128, 129, 130, 132, 133, 136, 137
fMRI data, 35, 36, 66, 69, 88, 105, 106
FMRIB Software Library (FSL), 7, 36, 37, 69, 107
forceps major, 37
forceps minor, 37
four repeats in the microtubule-binding domain (4R-tau), 53
fractional amplitude of low frequency fluctuation (fALFF), xi, xii, xvi, xvii, 2, 7, 16, 18, 37, 65, 99, 100, 104, 106, 107, 112, 113, 115, 124
fractional anisotropy (FA), ix, xv, 3, 32, 37, 43, 47, 49, 53, 54, 93, 97, 98, 102

fractional occupancy, 100
frame displacement (FD), 37
FreeSurfer, 69
frequency, xi, 3, 20, 64, 68, 69, 72, 76, 78, 81, 92, 97, 101, 108, 110, 119, 120, 124, 131
frontal, viii, xiv, 3, 8, 9, 10, 13, 14, 31, 33, 38, 39, 40, 41, 42, 43, 44, 46, 48, 51, 52, 53, 71, 72, 84, 85, 100, 101, 102, 103, 112, 113, 114, 116, 120, 121, 122, 124, 125, 126, 129, 135, 136
frontal cortex, ix, xiv, 32, 33, 71, 84, 112, 116, 122, 129
frontal lobe epilepsy, 101
frontal pole, 14, 38, 39, 40, 42, 48
frontal-cerebellum, ix, xv, 32, 43, 44, 52
frontoparietal, vii, xiii, xv, 1, 2, 5, 32, 33, 64, 68, 100, 101, 102, 103, 106, 125
frontoparietal atrophy, 33
frontoparietal network (FPN), vii, ix, xiii, xv, 1, 2, 5, 7, 9, 10, 11, 15, 16, 19, 20, 21, 32, 43, 44, 45, 52, 64, 68, 71, 73, 77, 78, 101, 106, 107, 109, 117, 118, 121, 124
frontoparietal region, 102, 103, 125
fronto-striatal, 3
frontotemporal dementia, 54, 55, 61
frontotemporal loss, 33
functional activation, 103
functional activity, xiii, 1, 2, 4, 20, 100
functional compensation, 2, 19, 20
functional connectivity, 2, 3, 5, 6, 19, 20, 24, 33, 37, 54, 66, 90, 91, 96, 100, 101, 103, 107, 109, 128, 129, 133
functional connectivity with MRI (fcMRI), 3, 37, 107
functional coordination, ix, xiv, 31, 34, 65
functional hubs, 107
functional mapping, x, 103
fusiform, 12, 14, 102

G

gender, 36, 71, 106
general AD-MCI, vii
genetics, 87
geometric distortion correction, 69
gliosis, viii, 32
global efficiency, viii, xiii, 1, 21, 53, 104, 115, 122, 123, 125
global signal, 68
globus pallidum, 40, 42
gradient-echo EPI, 6, 36, 105, 106
gradual volume reduction, 19
graph-theory, xi, xiv, 4, 7, 31, 34, 37, 53, 101, 104, 107, 115, 128, 134
gray matter atrophy, viii, xi, xiv, xvii, 6, 31, 32, 33, 38, 39, 51, 54, 99, 102, 112, 124, 125
gray matter density, xiv, 13, 14, 31, 33, 38, 39, 51, 112, 116
gray matter volume reduction, 33
group ICA of fMRI toolbox (Gift), 67, 68
group-ICA, 66

H

hallucination, x, 100, 103
hallucination severity, 103
hazard ratio, 3
hemodynamic function, 125
hippocampal atrophy, vii, xiii, 1, 7, 21
hippocampal occupancy (HOC), 71
hippocampal sclerosis, xi, 123, 125
hippocampal subfields, xii, 5, 19
hippocampal volume, 19, 71
hippocampus, vii, viii, xiii, xiv, 1, 2, 3, 5, 9, 11, 12, 13, 19, 21, 32, 38, 39, 40, 41, 47, 49, 51, 52, 85, 101, 102, 112, 121, 122, 129
hyper-synchronization, 66
hyper-synchrony, x, 101

hypo-connectivity, 34, 72, 73, 77, 78, 101, 103, 107, 109
hypothalamus, 9, 38, 39, 42

I

ICA-DR, viii, x, xi, xii, xv, xvi, 5, 7, 9, 10, 11, 15, 16, 17, 19, 20, 37, 43, 44, 45, 46, 52, 63, 65, 86, 88, 99, 104, 106, 120, 121, 124
ICA-DR algorithm, x, xii, xv, 7, 16, 19, 20, 52, 63, 86, 120, 121, 124
imaging abnormalities, vii, xi, xiii, xvi, 1, 4, 99
imaging differences, xii, xiv, 31, 34, 104, 124
imaging features, ix, xii, xv, 32, 34, 54
independent component analysis (ICA), viii, ix, xi, xii, xv, xvi, 2, 5, 7, 9, 10, 11, 15, 16, 17, 19, 20, 32, 37, 43, 44, 45, 46, 52, 63, 65, 67, 68, 71, 72, 86, 88, 91, 94, 99, 100, 104, 106, 107, 108, 120, 121, 124, 134
independent component analysis with dual regression (ICA-DR), viii, x, xi, xii, xv, xvi, 5, 7, 9, 10, 11, 15, 16, 17, 19, 20, 37, 43, 44, 45, 46, 52, 63, 65, 86, 88, 99, 104, 106, 120, 121, 124
independent vector analysis (IVA), 67, 94, 100, 127
inferior frontal gyrus (IFG), 3, 14, 20
inferior fronto-occipital fasciculus, 37, 43, 47, 49, 53
inferior longitudinal fasciculus, 37, 43, 47, 49, 53
inferior parietal lobe (IPL), 3, 9, 39, 44, 107
inferior parietal lobule, 104
information-based evidence, x
infratentorial structure, 34
insula, viii, x, xiv, 9, 31, 33, 40, 41, 52, 101, 102, 112, 124

insular network, 19
interhemispheric conductivity, x, xvi, 2, 19, 64, 86, 88, 100, 102
interhemispheric correlation(s), viii, xiv, 31, 40, 41, 42, 52, 54, 113, 121, 122
interhemispheric dis-coordination, vii, xiii, 1, 21
interictal epileptiform discharges, 101
inter-network connectivity, vii, ix, xiii, xiv, 1, 20, 21, 31, 32, 34, 43, 44, 52, 66, 102, 120, 121
inter-network correlation, 73, 118
inter-network dis-coordination, x, xvi, 64, 86, 88
inter-network hypo-connectivity, xi, xvi, 99, 123
inter-network modulation, x, xv, 63, 86, 124
inter-regional dependence, 101
intra-DMN, 8, 10, 19
intra-network variability, 66
intrinsic neuronal activity, 65

J

juvenile myoclonic epilepsy, 101, 129

K

k-means cluster, 67, 68
k-means clustering, 68

L

language, vii, xvi, 3, 64, 66, 70, 79, 82, 83, 86, 103, 133
language network, 103
large-scale networks, x, xv, 63, 65, 67
lateral occipital, 12, 13, 14, 38, 39
lateral occipital cortex, 14, 38, 39

leucine-rich glioma inactivated (LGI) family gene, 125
limb apraxia, viii, 33
lingual, 9, 12, 13, 14, 38, 39, 88, 102
lingual gyrus, 88, 102
local efficiency, viii, xiii, 2, 21, 48, 50, 51, 53, 115, 122, 123
local neuronal resources, 20
local relative efficiency, 17, 18
longitudinal change, 11, 12, 19, 104
longitudinal follow-ups, 66
longitudinal monitoring, 4
longitudinal prediction, 5
low frequency (LF), 16, 18, 72, 108, 110, 113
low-frequency synchrony, viii, xiii, 2, 21
low-sparsity level, 17, 18

M

magnetoencephalography (MEG), 101, 128, 134
major depressive disorder, 88
Markov chain modeling, 67
Markov modeling, ix, 65, 68, 100
MATLAB, 69
maximal mutual information, 67
MCI in general Alzheimer's disease (AD-MCI), vii, 3
MCI in Parkinson's disease (PD-MCI), vii, xiii, 1, 2, 3, 4, 5, 6, 7, 13, 14, 15, 16, 17, 18, 20, 21, 27
MCI in PD (PD-MCI), vii, xiii, 1
MD-MCI, 2
mean diffusivity (MD), 2, 37, 48, 49, 96, 97
mean dwell time, 68
medial prefrontal cortex (MPFC), 3, 8, 9, 10, 15, 16, 40, 42, 76, 77, 100
medial temporal atrophy index, 71
medial temporal lobe, 105

memory, xvi, 19, 20, 25, 64, 70, 79, 82, 83, 86, 132, 137
microscopic confirmation, 126
midbrain, 33, 40, 41, 42, 52, 56, 60
middle temporal gyrus, 33
mild cognitive impairment (MCI), vii, xi, xii, xiii, xvi, 1, 2, 3, 4, 5, 6, 7, 8, 9, 10, 11, 12, 13, 15, 16, 17, 18, 19, 20, 21, 22, 23, 24, 27, 35, 64, 66, 69, 70, 79, 81, 82, 83, 86, 91
mini-mental state examination (MMSE), 2, 20, 22, 23
molecular imaging, 21, 33
molecular underpins, 126
Montreal cognitive assessment (MoCA), 2, 6, 20, 22, 23
Montreal neurologic institute (MNI), 37, 68
mood, 20
morphological analysis, 6
morphological atrophy, 54
motion correction, 37, 70, 106
motion parameters, 68
motion restriction, 35, 36, 38, 48
motor, vii, viii, xi, xiv, 3, 5, 6, 8, 9, 10, 11, 13, 14, 15, 17, 19, 20, 26, 27, 31, 33, 34, 38, 39, 40, 41, 42, 43, 44, 45, 46, 51, 52, 64, 68, 98, 100, 103, 106, 112, 113, 116, 120, 121, 122, 124
motor area, 15, 20, 33, 40, 42, 52, 112, 113, 116, 121
motor coordination, 20
motor disorder, vii, 3, 20
motor network (MN), vii, xiii, 1, 3, 8, 9, 10, 11, 19, 26, 43, 44, 64, 66, 68, 71, 73, 77, 78, 86, 96, 106, 107, 108, 109, 117, 118, 124, 126
motor tract, 33
motor-related, 51
MPRAGE, 6, 36, 37, 105, 106
MRI, ix, x, xii, xiii, xv, xvi, 4, 6, 7, 31, 32, 34, 35, 36, 51, 53, 54, 55, 56, 60, 64, 69, 70, 71, 79, 82, 83, 84, 85, 86, 89, 95, 96, 103, 105, 106, 129, 131, 137
MRI regional volumetry, xii
MRI volumetry, 84, 85
MRI/PET, 4, 35, 137
multi-domain (MD), vii, 2, 20, 37, 48, 49, 51, 96, 97
multi-domain brain abnormalities, 51
multi-domain deficits, 20
multimodal, 4, 27, 53, 55, 56
multi-modalities, 101
multiomic features, xiii, 1, 4
multiomics, 21
multiparametric perspectives, xvii, 100, 126
multi-regional connectivity, 20
multivariate decomposition method, ix, 65
multivariate Gaussian and Laplace component vectors (IVA-GL), 67
myoclonus, viii, 33

N

National Alzheimer's Coordinating Center (NACC), 70
negative symptoms, 103
neocortex, viii, 32
neocortical focal epilepsy, 101, 129
neonates, 87, 97
network connectivity, ix, xiv, 5, 7, 8, 16, 19, 32, 33, 34, 43, 44, 52, 72, 88, 92, 94, 98, 119, 124, 127
network failure quotient (NFQ), 5, 7, 8
network modification, 125
network rerouting, 20
neurobiological model, 125
neurodegeneration score, 53
neurodegenerative diseases, xiii, 31, 34, 137
neurofibrillary tangles, 53
neuroimaging metrics, xiv, 31, 34

Index

NeuroImaging Tools & Resources Collaboratory (NITRC), xii, 104, 105, 127
neurological disease(s), x, xi, 4, 101
neuronal activity, x, 101
neuronal loss, viii, 32, 53
neuronal networks, xi, 123
neuropathological disease mechanism, ix, xv, 32, 54
neuropathological findings, 67
neuropathological mechanism, 19
neuropathology, viii, 32, 53, 96
neuropsychiatric disorder, x, 100
Neuropsychological batteries, 70
NeuroQuant (NQ), 71
neuroscience, x, 67, 137
nonamnestic deficits, vii, 2
normal control(s) (NC), vii, ix, xiii, xiv, 1, 2, 3, 5, 7, 8, 9, 10, 11, 12, 19, 21, 31, 35, 38, 39, 40, 41, 42, 43, 44, 48, 50, 53, 79, 81, 82
normal states, x, 67
novel imaging findings, 67
number of transitions, 101
nutrition, 20, 28

O

occipital lobe, 102
occipital pole, 14
occipitotemporal conjunction, 112
occupancy, 64
occurrence, x, xi, 68, 69, 74, 75, 78, 79, 80, 96, 108, 111, 119, 120
olfactory function improvement, 20
orbitofrontal cortex, 10, 48
orbitofrontal region, 40, 42, 52
overall dynamics, xi, xvi, 75, 80, 99, 108, 111, 123

P

palsy, viii, 33, 57, 58, 59, 60, 62
parietal, viii, xiv, 9, 10, 11, 12, 13, 19, 20, 31, 38, 39, 40, 41, 43, 44, 46, 51, 52, 71, 84, 85, 88, 100, 108, 113, 114, 121, 122, 124, 126
parietal cortex, 71, 84
parietal lobe, viii, xiv, 31, 40, 41, 52, 122, 124
parietal lobule, 88
Parkinson's symptom, viii, 32
Parkinson's disease (PD), vii, xi, xii, xiii, xiv, xv, xvi, 1, 2, 3, 4, 5, 6, 7, 13, 14, 15, 16, 17, 18, 20, 21, 27, 31, 33, 34, 54, 63, 64, 66, 67, 86, 130
Parkinson's progression markers initiative (PPMI), 5
Parkinsonism, viii, 23, 24, 28, 33, 34, 55, 62, 88
parsorbitalis, 11, 12
partial volume correction, 70
path length, 16, 18, 102, 115
pathway distortion, x, xvi, 64, 86
patient cohorts, x, xi, xiii, xiv, xvi, 31, 34, 64, 86, 99, 104, 123, 124
patient management, 54
pattern recognition, xv, 63, 67
PD with dementia (PDD), vii, 2, 3, 20
PD with MCI patients, xiv, 6, 13, 14, 17, 18, 31, 34, 66
PD without MCI, vii, xii, xiii, 1, 6, 13, 16, 18, 21, 66
PD-MCI, vii, xiii, 1, 2, 3, 4, 5, 6, 7, 13, 14, 15, 16, 17, 18, 20, 21, 27
PD-no MCI, 3, 4, 14, 20
pediatric epilepsy, 103
percentage of occurrence, 74, 75, 78, 80, 108, 110, 119
performance prediction, 4
perfusion-weighted imaging (PWI), 70

pericalcarine, 12, 76, 77
PET amyloid accumulation, xii
PET/MRI, xv, 32, 63, 64, 126
phenotypic harmonic score, 64
physical training, 20
physiological experiments, 127
physiological origin, 65
physiologically unconscious, viii, xii, xiv, 32, 35, 38, 64
pons, 42, 43, 47, 60
positive and negative syndrome scale (PANSS), 100, 102
positive symptoms, 102
positron emission tomography (PET), xii, xiii, xv, 4, 31, 32, 33, 34, 35, 56, 59, 63, 64, 69, 70, 71, 84, 85, 96, 126
post-central area, 11, 12
postcentral gyrus, x, 102
posterior cingulate, 3, 8, 10, 19, 71, 84, 100
posterior cingulate cortex (PCC), 3, 100
postural instability, 34
power spectrum, 68, 72
praxis, vii, 3
precuneus, 8, 9, 11, 12, 71, 84, 103
premotor, viii, xiv, 13, 14, 31, 33, 51
preprocessed functional data, 68
preseizure state, 103
prevalence, vii, 2, 20, 27
probabilistic tract template, 37
probable AD (pAD), 4, 5, 7, 8, 19
probable Alzheimer's disease (pAD), xiii, 1, 5, 7, 8, 19
progression, vii, 2, 4, 5, 19, 20, 23, 28, 35, 58, 69
progressive supranuclear palsy (PSP), v, viii, x, xi, xii, xiv, xv, 31, 32, 33, 34, 35, 38, 39, 40, 41, 42, 43, 45, 46, 47, 48, 49, 50, 51, 52, 53, 54, 56, 57, 58, 59, 60, 61, 62, 63, 64, 67, 69, 71, 72, 73, 74, 75, 76, 77, 78, 79, 80, 81, 86, 88, 91, 126
psychopathy traits, 87, 97
psychosis, xi, 125, 130, 135

putamen, 3, 33, 38, 39, 40, 42, 121, 122

Q

quality control, 71
quality of life, 21, 54
quantitative EEG (qEEG), 3, 26

R

radial diffusivity (RD), ix, xv, 3, 32, 37, 47, 49, 59, 93
rapid eye movement, 66
rare/comorbid cases, xii
realignment, 68, 70
recovery, 87, 97
red nucleus, viii, xiv, 32, 40, 41, 52
reference image, 6, 36, 105, 106
region of interest (ROI), 69, 71, 79, 81, 83, 86, 116, 117
regional homogeneity (ReHo), xi, xii, xvi, xvii, 99, 100, 104, 106, 112, 113, 114, 115, 122, 124
regional volumetry, 71
regional weighting, xi, xvii, 99
rehabilitation strategy, 4
relapsed psychosis, x, 100
relaxing condition, 105, 106
Religious Orders Study and the Memory and Aging Project (ROS/MAP), 70
removal of nuisance signals, 68
resting state (RS), viii, x, xii, xiv, xv, 31, 35, 36, 38, 39, 40, 41, 42, 43, 44, 45, 46, 48, 50, 51, 52, 53, 62, 63, 65, 67, 68, 69, 71, 72, 73, 76, 77, 78, 80, 81, 86, 88, 90, 93, 103, 105, 106, 117, 118, 126, 130, 136
resting state eyes closing (RS EC), viii, x, xii, xiv, xv, 31, 35, 38, 39, 40, 41, 43, 44, 45, 48, 50, 51, 52, 53, 63, 69, 71, 72, 73, 76, 77, 78, 86, 88

resting state physiologically unconscious (RS PH), viii, x, xii, xiv, xv, 31, 35, 38, 39, 40, 42, 43, 46, 48, 51, 52, 53, 63, 69, 76, 77, 78, 79, 80, 81, 86, 88
resting-state (RS)-fMRI, 6, 36, 105
resting-state fMRI, 32, 64, 89, 97, 103, 132
resting-state functional connectivity (RSFC), 2, 7, 19, 20, 37, 89, 100, 107, 133
reversal patterns, xi, xvi, 99, 123
reward-emotion circuit, 101
risk factors, 3, 7
rostral middle frontal area, 11, 12

S

salience network (SN), x, xi, xv, 9, 44, 63, 64, 68, 71, 73, 77, 78, 86, 87, 103, 106, 107, 109, 117, 118, 124, 125, 126, 128
salience-executive control network connectivity, 34
schizophrenia, v, x, xi, xiii, xvi, 66, 88, 91, 92, 93, 94, 97, 99, 100, 102, 104, 105, 106, 107, 108, 109, 110, 111, 112, 113, 114, 115, 116, 117, 119, 122, 123, 124, 125, 126, 127, 128, 129, 130, 131, 134, 135, 136
searching core nodes, 101
seed-based, 6, 19, 37
segmentation, 2, 71
segregation and integration, 101, 128
seizure frequency, 101, 104
seizure onset zone, 101, 103, 132
seizure propagation, 103, 125
seizure spread, 125
seizure(s), x, 100, 101, 103, 104, 105, 125, 132, 134
sensorimotor, 7, 9, 38, 39, 43, 45, 52, 66, 87, 102, 130
sensorimotor areas, 87
sensorimotor network, 7, 9, 66

significance levels, xvii, 99
simultaneous EEG-fMRI, 101, 125, 126
sliding-window(s), 65, 66, 67, 74, 89
slow wave bands, 113, 115
slow-wave, 16, 18, 66
slow-wave activity, 66
small-worldness, ix, xi, xiii, xiv, xv, xvi, 1, 7, 16, 18, 31, 32, 33, 34, 37, 48, 50, 51, 53, 99, 101, 104, 106, 107, 112, 115, 122, 123, 124
small-worldness analysis, xiii, 1, 16, 18, 37, 53, 101, 106, 115, 124
small-worldness configuration, 102
small-worldness factor, 17, 18, 48, 50, 53, 115, 122, 123
somatosensory, 8, 10, 38, 39, 40, 41
spatial concordance, 100, 103
spatial maps, 68, 117
spatial pattern, 65, 72
spatial resolution, 6, 36, 37, 105, 106
spatial smoothing, 68
spatial spreading, ix, xiv, 32, 38, 39, 40, 42, 52
spatiotemporal communication, xvi, 64, 86
spatiotemporal dynamics, 101
spectrum, xi, 3, 72, 117
speech and executive dysfunction, 34
spike correction, 66
spin-echo EPI, 37
SPM, 70, 116
standard composite scores, 70
standardized uptake value ratio (SUVR), 71, 84, 85
state, ix, xi, xii, xiv, xvi, 2, 22, 23, 25, 32, 35, 36, 38, 45, 57, 64, 65, 66, 67, 72, 73, 74, 77, 78, 86, 87, 89, 90, 93, 94, 97, 99, 102, 107, 108, 109, 110, 118, 119, 126, 127, 128, 132, 133, 134
state-based, xii, 67
state-based evidence, 67
state-dependent fluctuations, 66
state-shifting, xvi, 126

state-shifting role, xvi, 126
state-specific, 126
static functional connectivity, 100
static network analysis, x, 65
statistical comparisons, 38, 106
statistical correlation map, ix, 64
statistical validity, 65
striatum, xiv, 3, 31, 38, 39, 40, 42, 51, 121, 124
stroke, 87, 97
structural DTI alterations, 54
structural dysconnectivity, 54
structural integrity, viii, xiv, 31, 54
structural MRI, 36, 61, 70, 95
subcortical pathology, 53
subcortical regions, viii, xiv, 31, 38, 39, 42, 51, 52, 103
subfields, 5, 7, 19
subiculum (SUB), 5
substantia nigra, vii, xiii, 1, 3, 13, 20, 21, 40, 41, 53
subthalamic nucleus, 38, 39, 40, 41, 42
summation of pain, 87
superior frontal, vii, viii, xiii, xiv, 1, 11, 12, 13, 14, 19, 21, 31, 33, 38, 39, 40, 41, 42, 43, 44, 45, 48, 51, 52, 104, 113, 121, 122
superior frontal area, 40
superior frontal cortex, viii, xiv, 31, 40, 43, 44, 48, 52
superior frontal gyrus, 14, 33, 104
superior fronto-occipital fasciculus, 34
superior longitudinal fasciculus, 37, 48, 49, 102
superior longitudinal fasciculus (temporal part), 37, 48, 49
superior parietal lobe, 112
supplementary motor area (SMA), viii, xiv, 13, 14, 33, 38, 39, 43, 44, 46, 51, 52, 104, 120, 121, 122
supranuclear, viii, 33, 57, 58, 59, 60, 62
supratentorial microglial activation, 34
surgical guidance, 125

surgical intervention, x, 103
swallow tail sign, 13, 20
synchronizability, 104
synchronization, 93, 94, 101, 129
synchrony, 106, 113

T

TAR DNA-binding protein (TDP), 33, 53
tau burden, 11, 12, 33, 53, 56
tau deposition, viii, 12, 19, 32, 33
tau isoforms, 54
tau pathologies, 34, 61
tau plaques, 33
tau propagation, 53
tau tangle deposition, 11
tauopathy, 32, 36, 53
template space, 38
temporal, vii, viii, ix, xi, xiii, xiv, xv, 1, 7, 9, 10, 11, 12, 13, 14, 15, 16, 19, 21, 31, 38, 39, 40, 41, 42, 43, 44, 45, 46, 48, 51, 52, 63, 64, 67, 68, 71, 72, 84, 85, 86, 87, 88, 89, 91, 93, 100, 101, 102, 103, 104, 112, 113, 114, 116, 120, 121, 122, 123, 124, 125, 126, 128, 129, 132, 133, 134, 136
temporal cortex, 9, 15, 16, 19, 40, 42, 71, 84, 112
temporal dynamic(s), x, xv, 63, 64, 67, 86, 88
temporal gyrus, 14, 102, 116, 125, 129
temporal ICA, 68
temporal lobe, viii, xi, xiv, 32, 40, 41, 48, 52, 100, 101, 103, 104, 113, 114, 123, 124, 125, 126, 128, 129, 132, 133, 134
temporal lobe epilepsy (TLE), 101, 103, 104, 124, 128, 129, 132, 133, 134
temporal states, 68
temporal variation, ix, 64, 101
temporal vectors, 68
temporoparietal loss, 33
temporoparietal volume, xvi, 64, 86

test-retest reliability, 65, 90
thalamocortical, 5, 9, 43, 44, 45, 52, 66, 100, 102, 103, 121
thalamocortical anticorrelation, 66
thalamocortical connectivity, 5, 102
thalamocortical dysfunction, 100
thalamus, x, xiv, 8, 11, 13, 16, 31, 33, 38, 39, 40, 42, 51, 88, 102, 103, 113, 116, 117, 121, 122, 123, 124
therapeutic assessments, 4
Therapeutic Research Institute, 22, 71
time courses, ix, 64, 68
time series, ix, 64, 106, 129
total intracranial volume (ICV), 5
track-specific quantification, 47
tract-based spatial statistics (TBSS), 37, 43, 47
tract-based structural connectivity, xiv, 31, 34
tract-specific, 37
transient quantification, 125
transit changes, 87
transit interactions, 65
traumatic brain injury (TBI), 66, 92
treatment outcome, 87
tremor, 6
typical imaging, xii, 69, 88, 102, 112, 124
typical imaging findings, 88
typical MCI in general Alzheimer's disease (AD-MCI), vii, 2
typical Parkinson's disease, 33, 54
typical PD, xiv, 31, 34
typical symptoms, viii, 33

U

uncinate fasciculus, ix, xv, 32, 37, 47, 49, 53, 102
unified Parkinson's disease rating scale (UPDRS), 6, 20

V

variability of dFNC, 66
vascular malformations, 125
ventral striatum, 38, 39
ventromedial thalamic area, 112
vertical supranuclear gaze palsy, 34, 61
vigilance state, 66
visual, vii, viii, xi, xiv, 2, 5, 8, 9, 11, 13, 15, 19, 20, 31, 34, 38, 39, 40, 41, 42, 43, 44, 45, 46, 51, 52, 64, 66, 68, 72, 87, 100, 101, 102, 103, 106, 113, 114, 116, 120, 121, 122, 124, 130
visual attention, 20
visual cortex, viii, xiv, 13, 19, 20, 31, 38, 39, 40, 42, 51, 114
visual network (VN), xi, 9, 44, 64, 68, 71, 72, 73, 76, 77, 78, 86, 101, 106, 107, 109, 118
visual spatial, vii, 2
visual-motor, ix, xiv, 32, 43, 44, 45, 46, 52
visuospatial processing, 70, 79
vitamin D, 20, 28
VMHC deficits, xi, xvii, 99, 124
volumetry, 5, 7, 64, 84, 96
voxel mirrored homotopic correlation (VMHC), viii, x, xi, xii, xiv, xvi, xvii, 7, 13, 14, 19, 32, 37, 40, 41, 42, 48, 52, 86, 88, 99, 102, 104, 106, 112, 113, 121, 122, 124
voxel-based morphometry (VBM), xi, xii, xvi, 2, 7, 13, 32, 36, 37, 38, 39, 57, 99, 100, 102, 104, 105, 106, 112, 116, 124, 130
voxel-mirrored homotopic correlation (VMHC), viii, x, xi, xii, xiv, xvi, xvii, 2, 7, 13, 14, 19, 32, 37, 40, 41, 42, 48, 52, 86, 88, 99, 100, 102, 104, 106, 112, 113, 121, 122, 124

W

weighted inter-module normalization fractions, 5
white matter, ix, x, xv, xvi, 3, 25, 32, 33, 37, 54, 64, 86, 88, 102, 113, 114, 116, 117, 126, 130, 131
white matter deterioration, 33
white matter dysconnectivity, 126
white matter integrity, 3, 54
white matter integrity deterioration, 54
white matter skeleton, 37
window size, 65
within-cluster to between-cluster dissimilarity, 67

Z

z-score, 106